LOVE, CARE, & ALZHEIMER'S

A Daughter's Memoir

BING DEMPEWOLF

Copyright © 2024 by Bing Dempewolf

All rights reserved.

No part of this publication may be reproduced, distributed, or transmitted in any form or by any means, including photocopying, recording, or other electronic or mechanical methods, without the prior written permission of the publisher, except as permitted by U.S. copyright law.

For privacy reasons, some names, locations, and dates may have been changed.

Book Cover by Jolina Chan

ISBN: 978-1-7353895-8-5 (print)
ISBN: 978-1-7353895-9-2 (ebook)

For inquiries, please contact the author directly at:
bdempewolf@tai-chiconsulting.com

To my beloved mother, whose strength, wisdom, and love shaped my life. Though Alzheimer's tried to steal our memories, it could never erase the bond we shared. This book is for you, in honor of the woman who taught me the meaning of grace and unconditional love. May your light continue to shine in all that I do.

You remain forever in my heart.

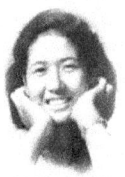

Content Statement

This memoir contains stories that address sensitive topics, including, but not limited to, child abuse and suicide. If you feel these potentially disturbing topics might be triggering, please consider your well-being before proceeding to read this book. For support, please dial 988 for the suicide and crisis lifeline.

Author's Note

To write this memoir, I relied on my memories to recount the events in this book. I didn't intend for the scenes and descriptions in this book to be word-for-word reenactments, nor are the events in chronological order. The dialogue is also not word for word but written to capture the spirit of the moment. I have also changed the names of some individuals for privacy reasons.

Spending over sixteen years caring for someone is hard to condense into a readable account. I could have written a thousand pages about everything that happened from the time of Mom's diagnosis to her death. To keep this memoir from becoming too repetitive, I did my best to choose key moments from my experience as a daughter and caregiver—snapshots of my mom's final years living with Alzheimer's.

Also, I want to stress that I am not a trained counselor or dementia expert. This is simply my recounting of my experience as my mom's caregiver during her sixteen-year journey with Alzheimer's. The resources I provide in this book were helpful to me, and I wish to share them with you.

For more information about dementia and Alzheimer's, please visit the Alzheimer's Association at https://www.alz.org.

Acknowledgements

First and foremost, I would like to express my deepest gratitude for the opportunity to share my journey with each one of you reading this book. I hope this provides some hope and encouragement when things get tough and you feel alone. Please know, you are not alone.

To Kevin, I could have never taken care of Mom at home without you. Your patience, understanding, incredible support, and constant love was the greatest source of strength to caring for Mom at home. Thank you from the bottom of my heart. To my children, Mike (Amy), Jon (Nicole), Lauren, Anthony, Kaden, and Kameryn, thank you for your support and for being a source of endless joy and motivation. Your smiles, laughter, and boundless energy have kept me grounded and focused, even on the most challenging days.

To Lauren, thank you for your love and dedication with taking care of Paw Paw and helping me through the different stages of her AD journey. You're an extremely special loving daughter/granddaughter for your love and support.

To Kaden and Kameryn, thank you for the love, patience, support, and encouragement to take care of Paw Paw at home and for understanding why we took care of her at home. For understanding why we didn't get to do a lot of things because she couldn't be by herself when was bedridden. You gave her the sparkle in her eyes when she saw you guys.

To my grandchildren, Conner, Brianna, Andre, Maelynn, Jonathan Jr., Max, Jessiah, Charlie, and Fitz, thank you for your love and support for your Tai-Paw.

To my siblings, Mon(Joe), Ning (Joanne), and Wai (Pam), thank you for your encouragement, support, and for always being there when I needed a listening ear or a word of advice. Your love and support mean the world to me.

To my niece and her family, Tasha, Carlos, Reagan, and Makenna, I extend my heartfelt gratitude for your unwavering support and encouragement throughout the journey of writing this book.

To my nephew, Michael and his amazing wife, Janet, thank you for your steadfast support and encouragement. Your kindness, understanding, and enthusiasm have been a true source of motivation.

To my nephew and his family, Brandon, Lacey, Cali, and Carter, thank you for your love and support for your AhMa.

To my staff, thank you for the support throughout the years Mom was sick. Each of you always made sure the business ran smoothly when Mom was in the hospital. I am deeply grateful for the countless hours you devoted to helping me when Mom needed me.

I would like to express heartfelt gratitude to Denise McGrail, whose talent and dedication as a ghostwriter made this project possible. Her ability to bring my ideas to life with clarity, creativity, and precision was invaluable. Denise, your collaboration, patience, and professionalism throughout this journey have been greatly appreciated. Thank you for your hard work and commitment to making this a reality.

I would like to thank Karen Tucker for your guidance, support, and belief in this project, and for being instrumental in publishing this book. Your editorial insights and expertise have made this journey an incredible experience. I am truly grateful for your dedication, professionalism, and partnership.

I am deeply grateful to Jolina Chan for creating the beautiful cover of this book. Your talent, creativity, and unwavering support have truly made my life better. You are a true blessing as my friend, always ready to help with dedication and grace. This book wouldn't have been complete without your incredible artistic contribution.

I am extremely grateful to Ron, whose unwavering love, support, and generosity made the dream of writing this book become a reality. Thank you for believing in me and my vision of this book. Your financial support provided me with the resources and freedom to make this book go from a dream to a reality. Beyond the financial aspect, your love, encouragement, patience, and understanding have been invaluable. You stood by me through the highs and lows, always offering a reassuring word and a helping hand. Your faith in my abilities game me the confidence to pursue this dream. Thank you from the bottom of my heart.

To all my family and friends, this book would not have been possible without each and every one of you. I am profoundly grateful for your contributions and for being a part of this journey with me.

Foreword

In the tapestry of life, some threads intertwine so seamlessly that they become inseparable, creating patterns of strength, resilience, and profound beauty. Such is the story woven by Bing Dempewolf in her poignant memoir *Love, Care, and Alzheimer's: A Daughter's Memoir*.

I first met Bing twenty-five years ago when she was the HR Director at our IT consulting firm. Little did I know then that this professional encounter would blossom into a friendship that would not only endure but flourish, intertwining our families and our lives in ways I could never have imagined.

As I write this foreword, I am struck by the parallels in our journeys. Like Bing, I too have walked the challenging path of caregiving. I first cared for my mother, Etta, during her struggle with lung cancer, and later for my father, Sebastian, as he battled an aggressive case of Alzheimer's. These experiences, while deeply personal, have given me a profound appreciation for the story Bing shares in these pages.

Bing's memoir is more than a mere recounting of events; it is a testament to the power of love, understanding, and cultural heritage. As an African American man reading about Bing's experiences in her Chinese American family, I was struck by the similarities in our cultures' approach to elder care. Both emphasize the importance of caring for our elders with vigor, compassion, and unwavering love. This shared value system, despite our different backgrounds, underscores the universality of filial devotion and the challenges that come with it.

What sets Bing's narrative apart is her remarkable ability to paint vivid pictures with her words. Her descriptive language creates a crisp backdrop for this intricate and complex love story between a mother and daughter, shaped by strict cultural norms. As readers, we are invited into a world where love is expressed not always through words or overt actions but through sacrifice, duty, and perseverance.

Bing's journey from feeling unloved to understanding and appreciating the depths of her mother's love is both heart-wrenching and inspiring. She masterfully portrays the complexities of growing up in a male-dominated culture, where her mother's love, though present, was often obscured by societal expectations and norms. The evolution of their relationship, culminating in Bing's dedicated care for her mother during the ravages of Alzheimer's, is a powerful reminder of love's ability to transcend cultural barriers and generational misunderstandings.

As someone who has witnessed the cruel progression of Alzheimer's firsthand, I can attest to the awe-inspiring dedication Bing demonstrated in caring for her mother. This awful disease tests the limits of both the patient and the caregiver, and Bing's unwavering commitment is a beacon of hope and strength for anyone facing similar challenges.

Over the years, Bing and I have recognized in each other kindred spirits—individuals who give freely of their time, talent, and treasure without expectation of return. This shared philosophy has led us to collaborate on numerous charitable endeavors and has shaped our approach to business and leadership.

Both Bing and I have embraced the principles of servant leadership throughout our careers as serial entrepreneurs. We believe in leading by example, putting the needs of others first, and using our success to uplift and empower those around us. This approach has guided not only our business ventures but also our philanthropic efforts.

Bing serves as the president of the board of directors for The Women's Safe House. Together with my wife Maria, I serve as an advocate against domestic violence on the executive board alongside Bing. When I was diagnosed with adult-onset blindness, Bing joined me on the board of directors for the St. Louis Society for the Blind and Visually Impaired. Our shared commitment to service has allowed us to be evangelists for the blind and visually impaired in the St. Louis metropolitan community.

These experiences have only deepened my admiration for Bing's resilience, compassion, and unwavering spirit—qualities that shine through every page of this memoir and have been evident in her approach to both business and philanthropy.

Love, Care, and Alzheimer's: A Daughter's Memoir is more than just a personal account; it is a universal story of love, duty, and the unbreakable bonds of family. It challenges us to look beyond surface-level expressions of affection and recognize the profound love that often manifests in sacrifice and steadfast care. Bing's narrative reminds us that even in the face of a disease that steals memories, the essence of love remains undiminished.

As you embark on this journey through Bing's memories and experiences, I invite you to open your heart to the lessons within. Let her words inspire you to cherish your loved ones, to seek understanding across generational and cultural divides, and to find strength in the face of life's most daunting challenges. Moreover, let her example of servant leadership inspire you to consider how you might use your own talents and resources to make a positive impact in your community and beyond.

In a world that often seems fragmented and divided, Bing's story is a powerful reminder of our shared humanity and the love that binds us all. It is a testament to the transformative power of servant leadership, both in business and in life. It is my honor to introduce you to this remarkable memoir and to the extraordinary woman behind it—a true servant leader whose impact extends far beyond the pages of this book.

-Kenneth L. Tabb
BBAT Enterprises, LLC

1

You're Stealing from Me!

Mom and I stood in my kitchen at the sink on a sunny day—one of those cloudless days when the sun is at its fullest and brightest, an instant mood booster. Nothing seemed out of the ordinary that day with Mom. Nothing that would've warranted her sudden outrage and the accusations that spewed from her lips.

"You're stealing from me!" she yelled at me.

"What?" I searched her face for signs she was joking. She had to be joking, right? I would never steal from her. But I found no playfulness in her eyes. What I saw shocked me more than her words because displayed all over her face was anger and betrayal.

I stood in shocked silence and disbelief for what seemed an eternity but was probably no more than a few seconds, trying to decide what to say and how to react.

"Mom," I said when I finally found my words, "no, I'm not stealing from you. I would never steal from you."

How could she think I would steal from anyone, much less my family? Over the last seven years, my husband, Kevin, and I had opened our home to her, taking care of her after my father died and tending to her various health issues. We gave her a place to live surrounded by family instead of being alone after forty years of marriage. We provided a safe, loving household for her, cooked meals for her, and had even bought her a car to drive. We had gone above and beyond to show Mom unconditional love and care. Why would I steal from her?

Her accusations landed in my gut like a hard punch, and they were still coming.

When she spoke again, her nostrils flared, and her eyes grew wide. She yelled, "You stole my credit card number!"

"No, I didn't steal from you, Mom," I said again, to no avail. I had to sit down to catch my breath as she continued to accuse me. Who knew words could literally knock the wind out of you?

"You thief! You're a liar! You're stealing my money," she kept insisting. Mom was raging, and I was crying. How could she say such awful things to me? Why was she being so hateful? Never in my life had I felt so hurt by her actions—and believe me, there were plenty of times Mom hurt me.

I sat at the kitchen table, frustrated and confused, my head in my hands. Tears trailed down my cheeks. I heard her feet shuffle across the kitchen floor and then her bedroom door close. I didn't dare glance in her direction.

A few moments later, while still sitting at the kitchen table with my head in my hands, I felt someone stroking my back. I looked up, expecting to see Kevin or one of my children. Instead, it was my mom. The person who'd *just* called me a thief and a liar.

"Why are you crying?" she asked. Her voice held none of the

fury it had hurled at me moments earlier. Instead, it was loving.

"What do you mean?" I asked, very confused and still reeling from her hurtful accusations. "I'm crying because you accused me of stealing from you. You said I stole your credit card number and have been taking your money."

She frowned at me and studied my face for signs that I was joking, not unlike how I reacted when she'd first accused me. Then she smiled and shook her head, gazing at me like I was a child making up a story.

"No, I didn't say that. You're my daughter. Why would I say that?" She continued to rub my back softly, her touch light and soothing. Then she smiled, told me she loved me, and walked away from the table.

I stared at her back as she walked away. I couldn't speak. Shock waves radiated throughout my body. *What just happened?* I thought. *Does she really have no memory of accusing me of stealing her money? How can she not remember how hateful she was to me? Had I imagined it?* I had been working long hours as a C-Suite executive. Maybe the work stress was catching up to me and I was seeing and hearing things.

Then the situation went from bad to worse. Over the following days, she called my siblings and told them I had stolen her credit card number and was taking her money. And, even more to my surprise, I got the impression my siblings believed her! They never came right out and said they believed her. They never accused me directly like Mom did, but the tone of their voices said otherwise. It was four against one. I felt defeated because I knew I hadn't stolen from my mom. But how could I prove to them I wasn't taking her money—and more importantly, why was she convinced I was?

The reason would become clearer as the days and weeks progressed, and I learned the true nature of Mom's memory lapses and behavioral changes. But at that moment, all I could feel was a jumble of emotions and incredibly alone, much like many caregivers caring for loved ones diagnosed with dementia and probable Alzheimer's disease (AD). Alzheimer's, like other types of dementia, does more than steal a person's memories. It steals their very essence. It steals time, and it steals sanity from both the diagnosed individual and that person's loved ones and caregivers. It's cruel. It's relentless. And it makes loved ones feel very much alone.

That's why I wanted to write this book. Right now, as I write these words, the World Health Organization (WHO) estimates there are fifty-five million people worldwide living with dementia. By the time this book reaches your hands, that number will have increased as approximately ten million new cases are diagnosed yearly. My story isn't unique, but so often, family members navigating dementia journeys with their loved ones feel isolated and unheard. They often recognize something is *off* with their loved one long before anyone else, and without answers, they often feel like they're losing their sanity.

Caring for my mother during her illness was a great honor, but I'd be misleading you if I said it was something I always felt compelled to do. I have always had a complicated relationship with my mom. Many children have complicated relationships with their parents that last well into adulthood. Mine started from birth. You see, as a first-generation Chinese American, I grew up in a household where my mom showed more respect for my brothers than me and my sister. It's how she was raised in China and how she raised us in America.

Mom wasn't an affectionate person, and she didn't outwardly show any sort of pride in me or my accomplishments. Her lack of affection forged a massive canyon between us, especially when she refused to intervene and protect me from my abusive father. For so long, I felt unloved and not taken care of. I couldn't let go of the anger and hurt that I felt—and then Mom became ill.

Long before her probable Alzheimer's diagnosis, she needed help. At first, it was to assist her in taking care of my dad, who had developed liver cancer and died six months after retiring. I quit a great job to stay with Mom and help her care for Dad. After he passed, I started worrying about her health problems. She had serious issues, like diabetes and failing kidneys. I also worried she might develop anxiety living alone. I wondered what it would look like if I became her caregiver. Would I care for her with love and compassion or resentment and hostility? As a Chinese American daughter, and the youngest at that, what duty did I owe her?

Caring for my mom was an emotional roller coaster, one that I had thought I was prepared to ride, but how prepared could I have been? I'd never experienced caring for someone with dementia, and when that person is a parent, it's a complex process because there's history. There's a backstory that is rarely sunshine and roses. The parent-child relationship is intricate and sometimes contentious. It's a relationship unlike any other, and when roles become reversed, it's more perplexing.

In this book, I share stories about my childhood and what it was like growing up in America with Chinese-born and -raised parents and how that affected my feelings toward my mom while caring for her for over two decades, sixteen of those years while she moved through the AD journey. Although my upbringing may differ from yours, if you have a parent diagnosed with AD or another form of dementia and didn't have the perfect relationship with your parent—Is there even such a thing?—I hope reading this book helps you feel less alone and your conflicting feelings more supported.

Throughout these pages, I take you on a journey with me. A journey no one wants to take because losing a parent to dementia is heartbreaking, and it's backbreaking when you give all of yourself to care for them. I don't regret taking care of Mom, but I gave up so much of myself to do that. I also gave up my family life. There were so many things I couldn't do with my kids because of my role as a caregiver. You probably feel the same way.

Perhaps you picked up this book because your loved one has recently received a diagnosis of dementia and you're seeking answers. I can't promise to have any answers for you. I'm not a medical professional, and I have no formal training in

Alzheimer's and dementia care. What I have is my story, and stories matter. They connect us and make us feel less alone. I hope as you read this story, you find a bit of yourself in it. I hope you find solace in knowing you're doing your best with the resources and energy you have. It's difficult to walk this journey with our loved ones. It's long and filled with twists and turns and lulls, and it has a predetermined ending. There's no surviving Alzheimer's. It gets you in the end, and it's merciless.

I hope as you read my story, you feel less alone and that you know it's okay to take care of yourself. Caregiving is exhausting, and caring for a loved one with AD or dementia is, most times, all-encompassing. Yet we find strength in unexpected ways, and from my experience, we develop a new relationship with our loved ones. In many ways, caring for a parent with dementia deepens the relationship and leaves us with a newfound sense of their life and struggles, and opens our hearts and eyes to seeing our parents in a different light.

There are so many things I probably could've done differently, but you only know what you know at the time, so have grace and be patient with yourself. You're doing the best you can.

2

New Beginnings

In September 1966, my parents, Chun Choi and Kwai "Bessie" Chiu, and my three older siblings, Monika (Mon), Ning, and Wai, immigrated to the United States from China to start a new life. Mom was three months pregnant with me when she and my dad found themselves living with his sister in St. Louis, Missouri. My aunt had sponsored my parents so they could leave China, which had become an increasingly controlling country since China's communist leader Mao Zedong created the People's Republic of China (PRC) in 1949. Dangerous, too. My grandparents had owned a small corner store in China and enjoyed a fair life, but the communists thought they had money and they weren't giving it up. So one day, they came for my grandparents. They took them from their store to the town center and murdered them. My parents' homeland was no longer welcoming or safe. It was time to leave.

Building a new life in a new country where my parents didn't speak the language was difficult, to say the least. My parents hadn't gained the complete independence they sought when moving to the United States because of their dependency on my aunt's family for food and shelter. They were treated like sub-class citizens and expected to work for free at the family's chop suey carryout restaurant. In China, Mom was a registered nurse and Dad was a pharmacist, but those credentials didn't matter here. If my parents wanted to work in their respective fields, they had to obtain their professional licenses in America. The problem wasn't their education or knowledge. It was the language barrier. Learning English proved difficult. It took Mom many years before she could overcome the barrier to receive her RN license, but my dad never received his pharmacy license. He couldn't overcome the language barrier like Mom, and even though he had over ten years of experience as a pharmacist in China, he only qualified to work as a pharmacy technician in his new homeland, earning a fraction of what he would've made as a pharmacist. A Chinese woman making more than her husband was not something a Chinese man would've taken lightly—and my father didn't.

The Chinese philosopher Confucius is well known for his statement that an "educated woman is a worthless woman." After all, Confucius believed a good woman was an illiterate one, and men in Confucian families were held to the highest esteem.

I was born in May of 1967 in America to immigrant Chinese parents who held many of the beliefs Confucius taught—specifically the importance placed on sons—and that caused a lot of tension and rifts in my relationship with my parents during my childhood. I remember during a turbulent time of my adolescence when I couldn't understand why we couldn't be that normal American family. The *Leave It to Beaver* family, who ate dinner together every night, talked about their day, and the children and parents had pleasant relationships with each other.

My childhood was nothing like that idealistic television show.

My dad was physically abusive. He believed wives (all females, actually) should be seen and not heard, and while Mom was on the receiving end of some of his abuse, the brunt of it fell on me and my older sister, Mon. The anger and frustration he felt about his situation he took out on Mon and me, or at least as an adult, that's what I assume was the source of his rage. I can't say for certain and, really, it doesn't matter. It doesn't change the fact that in his fits of rage, he would beat us with belts, hockey sticks, and orange plastic Hot Wheels tracks. If he didn't want us to leave, he'd bolt our doors with 2x4 wood pieces. Sometimes Mom would step in and try to protect us, but she was powerless and couldn't stand up to him. I see that now, but back then, I felt forsaken and confused. I couldn't understand why the two people who were supposed to love me more than life itself were hurting me, one physically and the other by turning away. I didn't know where to turn for help. Who would understand? My friends weren't Chinese. They wouldn't understand. I felt so alone and unloved.

The only person who could relate was Mon, but when she turned eighteen she moved out. With Mon gone, Dad's rage turned solely on me. I was eight years old and suffering severe child abuse from my dad while I felt my mom did little to stop it. The abuse continued for years. I hated my life, and I was depressed. I was a child. I was supposed to be playing with friends and living a life without worry. My parents were supposed to protect me. I had none of that. Instead, I was working in the family restaurant cleaning tables, serving food, and doing whatever was asked of me—all free labor except for the measly tips I earned, I should add.

The toll of living with daily abuse and what it did to my self-worth came to a head when I turned eleven. I couldn't take my life anymore and decided to end it—twice. My dad had a lot of back pain for which he took painkillers to relieve his discomfort. I found his painkillers and took a handful of them. A family friend found me, took me to the hospital, and I had my stomach pumped and things were fine. Well, not fine, but I was alive and then life just carried on. Things went back to normal, meaning daily abuse from my dad, Mom looking the other way, and me continuing to hate my life.

It wasn't long after my first suicide attempt that I attempted to take my life again. This time, I was nearly successful. I actually died on the table and had to be brought back to life. Mom was working as a nurse at Normandy Osteopathic Hospital in Normandy, Missouri, a St. Louis suburb, and was on duty when I was brought in after ingesting more of my dad's painkillers. Mom had been working on the second floor when one of her coworkers delivered the news.

"Bessie," she said, using Mom's American name, "your daughter's been brought into the emergency room. She took some pills. She coded, but the doctors brought her back."

Once I became a mother, I understood how frightening and

devastating that moment must've been for my mother. As angry, hurt, and confused as I was at eleven years old, taking my life was what I thought was the only way out of an abusive situation. To this day, I wish I'd never done that. I wish I'd never put my mom through the terror of not knowing if I was going to live or die. I still carry regret today because I know what I would've felt if one of my children had done what I did. Still, at that time, I felt like I had no other options because I felt isolated and my life was completely out of control. Suicide for an eleven-year-old should never be an option.

After the second suicide attempt, I didn't go home. Instead, my parents admitted me to a psychiatric hospital. It was hell.

Can you imagine being eleven years old and living in a psychiatric ward? If you've ever seen the 1999 film *Girl, Interrupted*, starring Angelina Jolie and Winona Ryder, you might get a glimpse of what life's like in a juvenile psychiatric ward. But let me tell you this, until you're in one, you can't possibly have any actual idea. If you're reading this and had a similar experience, my heart breaks for you. No child should have to endure the nightmare of a psychiatric hospital.

Let me paint you a picture of what it was like during my stay in 1978.

First, let's start with the word stay. It makes it sound like a getaway, a brief vacation to rest and get back on track. To fix what is wrong. That's hardly what a stay in a juvenile psychiatric ward is like.

First, they took everything from me. They took my

shoestrings and the sash to my robe. They didn't allow me to have anything that I could potentially harm myself with. Anger poured out of me like a spilled ink bottle, dark and thick. And because I was angry that my parents had sent me to this scary place, the staff assumed I was violent. Don't get me wrong. There were others in that psychiatric ward with me who were violent, but I wasn't. I was mad that my parents had tossed me aside, leaving me feeling abandoned, unloved, and unworthy. Once the staff made their assumptions about me, they took more of my autonomy and dignity. They put me in a straitjacket and tossed me in a padded room and only my mom visited me. She tried to come every day. My father never visited me.

No one cared about me in that place. The therapy offered wasn't helpful. No one asked me why I tried to kill myself. The staff didn't seem to want to get to the bottom of why I'd want to end my life. Living in America with a Chinese family was a dynamic most people, including the staff, struggled to understand. The staff's primary goal was to manage their patients, not treat them or help them come out stronger and healthier. Even our education wasn't a concern and it was more difficult because it wasn't offered in a traditional classroom setting. No one taught us anything. They gave us textbooks and expected us to figure out the lessons ourselves.

I wanted out so badly, but I also didn't want to go home. I couldn't go back to that situation. Mom might have shown up most days to visit, but I knew nothing had changed back home. If I went back there, the abuse would resume. I wanted to live with Mon, who had since moved out, but she was twenty-one and in college. She didn't want the responsibility of looking after her little sister. I didn't understand that as a child, but as an adult, I get it.

Surprisingly, between my second suicide attempt and my time in the psychiatric ward, Mom took action. She understood I couldn't live with my dad. So, she rented a house for me.

I know what you're thinking. What mother sends her daughter to live alone at eleven years old? I felt the same way for a long time. Though Mom did this to keep me safe (and it did essentially save my life), I didn't see it this way as a little girl. I felt abandoned and alone. I was a child and expected to work at our family restaurant and use the tips I made to pay my bills, including half the rent. Mom paid the other half. I resented her for years for how she treated me. It would take a long time, well into my adulthood, even up to the point of Mom's AD diagnosis, if I'm being truthful, until I came to understand she couldn't stay in the house with me because my father wouldn't have it. He didn't care where I was or what I was doing, but he cared if Mom wasn't home. So, as incredulous as it sounds, the solution she came up with was—I believe—the best she could do at the time for someone in her situation with an abusive husband, living in a new country, and learning its customs while trying to protect her child; although it would take me a long time to see her actions as protection or understand that the myriad reasons she left me alone didn't matter because she was doing the best she could for her child. The best is all we can hope for

for sometimes.

I didn't always live alone in the house. Mom actually intended for my older brother, Ning, who was twenty, to live with me. But he came and went as he pleased. Rarely did he come to the rental and stay with me. So, essentially, I lived alone until I was fourteen. That's when I met Mick.

Mick was my brother's friend, a twenty-three-year-old man who started paying attention to me. I couldn't believe this person liked me. To have someone finally paying attention to me felt amazing. After I spent my entire young life feeling alone, someone finally seemed to care.

My dad took notice too, but not the way you'd think a father would notice when a grown man is messing with a young girl. Dad took notice of Mick's job at a local Fortune 500 company specializing in engineering services for industrial, commercial, and consumer markets because in Chinese culture fathers looked for older males with good jobs who could provide for their daughters so they would no longer have this burden. A job at this particular company in the mid to late 1970s was prestigious and attractive to my father. Once he realized Mick's interest in me, my father saw a way to wash his hands of me. He took me to the St. Louis County Courthouse, where he obtained a marriage certificate for me because, at fifteen, I couldn't make that decision for myself—not that my consent mattered to my dad. Shortly after that, Mick and I married.

The only example of marriage I had was my parents' marriage.

I didn't know what to expect beyond that, but I thought it had to be better than the life I'd been living up to that point. Within a year of marriage, I was pregnant, and by the time I was twenty-two years old, I had four children. Many people thought my life was over, but I loved my children. I felt differently about my marriage. By the time I was twenty-five, my marriage had ended and for the better, because my marriage to Mick wasn't any better than the life I'd lived before. While I might have escaped my dad's abuse, I experienced emotional and physical abuse in my marriage. Mom always told me I must stay in the marriage, no matter what, but the thought of staying was scarier than leaving. So I did the unimaginable to some: I filed for divorce and became a single mother of four children.

It was a scary, uncertain time of my life, being so young and having four precious children depending on me. I had to be their role model and show them what we could do together. I lived in my car for a while because I couldn't live at home, but the kids wanted to be with me. I didn't want to live on the streets, dependent on government assistance. I didn't merely want us to survive; I wanted us to thrive. So, I pulled from my inner strength, a path that surprisingly came from my mom.

3

A Mother's Strength

Kwai "Bessie" Chiu was a tenacious woman, even if her strength and fortitude weren't always evident to me. I held much resentment in my heart toward my mom when I was a child and even into my early adulthood. As a young Chinese girl, I thought a lot about Barbie, the plastic doll, and the idealized world that surrounded the Barbie brand. I wanted that idealistic life (and the blonde hair), but life at home was nothing like it. I blamed my mom for my dad's abuse and couldn't wrap my mind around her lack of protection, but something happens when you become a parent. You gain a clearer understanding of the subtleties of parenthood. The world becomes more colorful, less black and white, and, if you allow yourself, you see your parents as more than caregivers and protectors. You see them as people who are flawed and struggling as much as you are.

Mom couldn't stand up to my dad. She was no match for his demons. But let me assure you this: Her protective love made its way to me the best it could. As an abused and silenced woman, she had to wield her protection under the radar. She made small, quiet moves that wouldn't upset my dad and, in the long run, kept me safer. As children, we don't understand the nuances of protection or a parent's love—and in this case, a mother's love.

We always hear people say they'd do anything for their children. *Anything.* But what does that really mean? Circumstances limit what you can do. There are plenty of people who hold an abused woman's choices against her. Why did you stay in a relationship that's hurting your children? Why didn't you leave? Couldn't you have done more?

I had those thoughts about Mom too. It was only by raising my young family that I saw her circumstances through a different lens. She did what she could with limited opportunities. Yes, my mom had a good job as a charge nurse, and once she'd overcome the language barrier and earned her RN license in this country, her earning potential gave her more opportunities. Still, her professional accomplishments didn't stop her from feeling beholden to my dad. Being raised in a traditional Chinese family planted deep-rooted beliefs in what it meant to be a wife. Living on American soil didn't change those beliefs. So, she worked with what she had. What she had was her education and her desire to provide whatever she could, in whatever manner was available to her, for her children.

And Mom worked hard.

Even when we didn't have a great relationship, I knew she worked hard to persevere. Anytime the chance to work overtime presented itself, she snagged it. She used the extra money to pay for my brother's education at Washington University in St. Louis, Missouri, and to help him get a car. She worked overtime to rent the "safe" house for me. Not only did she work full-time as a charge nurse, but she was an entrepreneur too. She started and successfully ran other businesses: Asian Imports, a store that sold knickknacks and tchotchkes, and a sit-down Chinese restaurant at the corner of Florissant and Lindbergh in north St. Louis County called Hong Kong Restaurant. I heard people complain when they had too much to do, but Mom never whined when her plate was full. She took life in stride, doing what she needed to do for herself and her children to thrive. She consistently had new ideas to make more money to support the family whenever someone needed something. But no matter how much success she seemed to achieve from an outsider's perspective, the truth was Mom was always ten steps behind her American friends and co-workers because when she went home at the end of the day, she walked through the front door to another culture where women were treated differently. Still, Mom worked with cultural limitations, parenting and supporting us the best she could, even when she had to play small and stay under the radar. Her quiet resilience has affected me greatly throughout the course of my life.

It's made me the woman I am today.

Having a baby at fifteen presented its challenges, especially when it came to completing my education. Like Mom, I wasn't going to let my circumstances derail the ambitions I had for myself. With a young child and little support, I could've resigned to the notion that having a family meant not having anything more. Still, I pushed for something better.

I enrolled in McCluer High School's Education Center, an

alternative education program. Some struggled with drug addiction, behavioral problems, and other issues that earned them the label of "misfits." Then there were the students like me—high-achieving students who had life circumstances that made it difficult to attend traditional high school classes.

This was the early 1980s. There weren't online courses I could take to complete the credits I needed to earn my high school diploma. Sure, I could've studied for the GED, but I wanted a truer high school experience, and I knew I could handle the coursework even with a new baby and home responsibilities—and I did. I completed the credits I needed to graduate within a year and a half, graduating at sixteen years old.

I credit much of my success at McCluer's Education Center to a teacher named Tom Beil, even though I had a strong dislike for him at the time. I might have been a young mother and living on my own (albeit with Mick), but that didn't mean the surly teenage behavior passed me over. Not at all. I hated Mr. Beil because he pushed me. He saw my potential, even when I couldn't see it myself.

"Why are you pushing me?" I'd say to him.

His response was to push me harder. He knew I was an educated kid. I wasn't a burnout. I know that term's outdated and cringy, glossing over behavioral and learning issues that many high school students struggle to overcome and leads them to making poor choices for themselves. But during the early 1980s, this is how many students in alternative education programs were thought of. Since that wasn't my situation, my teachers expected more, especially Mr. Beil. In a sense, he took the place of my parents and became an influential person in my young life. He wasn't the type of teacher who sat at a desk and regurgitated facts, expecting his students to memorize them, take a test, and call it done. No, Mr. Beil taught us how to be better students. The skills he taught prepared me for college, where you're expected to think critically and take control of your studies.

Mr. Beil not only pushed me to be the best student I could be, but he was there for me during a time when I was really depressed. His open-door policy and kindness toward me made it easy to talk to him, and he gave me strength when I couldn't always find it within myself. It's been over forty years since I sat in Mr. Beil's classroom, and to this day, I still consider him an important part of my formative teenage years.

Mr. Beil didn't quit on me, and Mom never quit on herself. The two most influential people in my life during my formative teenage years shaped my transition from childhood to motherhood. It was important to me to teach my children what Mom had taught me, directly and by implication. I had to be the role model they needed and, most importantly, deserved. With the image of Mom planted firmly in my mind, her strength and the proverbial wind at my back, I knew a high school diploma wasn't enough to thrive as a single mom. If my children and I were going to live beautiful lives teeming with opportunities, I had to have skills to make money—good money. So, I went to college, earning multiple degrees, including my MBA, all while working as many jobs as necessary to give my children everything they needed.

During this time, Mom and I were working toward mending our fractured relationship. I tried to forgive her for turning away from my dad's abuse, or at the very least, I tried to make peace with acceptance. Still there were times I wanted her to show up like the mothers of friends or even those on television. I yearned for her help with my four young children, but as an overnight nurse, watching her grandchildren was difficult for her. As much as I understood that, it still pained me that once again I felt very much alone.

After my divorce, I spent the subsequent years focusing on getting my education and earning my degrees and raising my children. I enjoyed the freedom that came from being unshackled from an abusive relationship and truly loved the life I was building for myself and my children. All the degrees in the world couldn't trump the feeling of providing a beautiful life for my children, a life I never quite had as a child. To this date, it's one of my proudest achievements. Caring for Mom during her battle with AD ranks a close second, but we'll get to that later.

Yet, even though I was mostly content and extremely busy during my twenties parenting, working, and going to school, something was missing. Loneliness carved a deep hole in my being. I yearned to find love, a partner who I could do life with. I tried dating, but it was hard with four kids. The men I met were interested in me but weren't keen on becoming a stepparent to four children under the age of thirteen. Could I blame them? Most men in their twenties are focusing on finishing school, starting their careers, and maybe thinking of marriage and children as they approach thirty. Finding a man who wanted a ready-made family from the first date proved nearly impossible. After many failed relationships, I decided to swear off men until my youngest, Anthony, was out of college.

Then I met Kevin.

Our meet-cute moment happened on a flight coming home from Chicago. I traveled a lot for work in the mid-90s and flew frequently, which meant I spent a lot of time away from my kids, and that particular day, I couldn't get to my kids fast enough. I had a first-class ticket for a later flight but gave it up for a standby position on an earlier one. At the last second, I got the standby seat and gracelessly made my way down the aisle with my overnight bag, laptop, and purse flopping about, searching for an empty seat. Fortunately, I found an aisle seat, but the overhead compartments were full. So, I asked the gentleman sitting in the middle seat (whom I would soon learn was named Kevin) if I could place my bag under his seat. He said sure and I sat down prepared for a quiet flight back home, but Kevin had other ideas.

Flying as much as I did, I met a lot of interesting people, and talking to people rarely bothered me. Still, I'd had a long day. The finish line to home was in sight, and I wanted to spend the next forty-five minutes to an hour in peace. But Kevin was a talker. I learned he worked off of Page and 270 in St. Louis County. I worked off Olive and 270. For those of you who aren't familiar with the St. Louis Metro area, what that meant is we were near each other, but I wasn't really interested in him romantically. He didn't seem my type—or the type my assistant thought I had: tall, dark, and handsome. The conversation wasn't bad though, and I figured if we were in the area together sometime that maybe we could catch up and have lunch or a drink. What could it hurt? We exchanged numbers.

A few weeks went by and a client stood me up for a meeting at Westport Plaza, a commercial development off 270 and Page that had dining, entertainment, and office spaces. I'm not sure what made me do it, other than curiosity or that I had a sitter I'd already paid to watch the kids, but I called him.

"Hey, are you busy?" I asked, surprised he picked up. "Would you be interested in dinner?"

Let's just say I didn't have to twist his arm. Actually, to my surprise, he confessed to me at dinner that he hurried home to change into nicer clothes before meeting up. No way was he showing up in the jeans he'd worn to work that day. That gave me pause in a good way. Sure, he wasn't the usual guy I dated, but most of those guys were jerks. There was one guy I dated when my kids were younger whom I met at Plaza Frontenac, an upscale mall in the St. Louis suburbs where you can spend a small fortune at Louis Vuitton, Gucci, and Tiffany & Co in one day if you desire and your bank account has plenty of zeros. The day I met him, he put down three hundred dollars on a pair of gloves.

"You know," I told him, "you can get similar gloves at Target for ten dollars."

Nonetheless, I let him take me to Cardwell's for dinner one night, an exclusive, classy restaurant that wasn't inexpensive. At this point, I might've shared my opinion about his spending habits, but I hadn't told him about my kids. Bringing up my kids to a potential suitor was tricky. Like I mentioned earlier, not many men were keen to date a woman barely thirty years old with four children, not to mention teenagers. I went back and forth with myself about whether to bring up my kids in conversation. Well, I brought them up. What happened next? Remember pagers in the '90s? This man had one and shortly after I told him about my kids, he pretended he got paged, left to return the nonexistent page, and never returned. I told you: Dating with kids was tricky.

But Kevin was different.

For starters, he was seven years older than me. He'd never been married and didn't have kids, but he seemed ready for a family—or, at least, a built-in family didn't scare him away. At that time in my life, with four children, I felt pulled in four different directions constantly. He wanted to help me and I let him. After all, I didn't know a thing about football and basketball that my sons were into. Having someone who could teach me and be a role model to my boys and my daughter, Lauren, too, was appealing. Maybe my initial attraction to Kevin was out of convenience, but he was the first man in my life who showed up in a real way for me. Little did I know then, during that first dinner date, how much Kevin, whom I eventually married, would support me throughout the years, especially when taking care of Mom.

4

What's Going on With Mom?

In June of 1998, my dad passed away and Mom, at sixty-five years old, had begun to battle several health challenges, including diabetes and failing kidneys. I worried about her living alone after forty-plus years of marriage. I thought her living alone would leave her anxious, but she insisted she'd be fine. Reluctantly, I let her be. It was hard for me to believe taking away her freedom was the right thing to do. What say did I have in how she lived her life? Little did I know at the time that Alzheimer's would eventually steal her freedom and so much more. But at that time, I yielded to her desire to live alone, all the while keeping a close eye on her to ensure her well-being.

It didn't take long for my fears of her living alone to come true.

Not long after my dad died, Mom, Kevin, and I made plans to go shopping. Before leaving our house, I called Mom to see if she was ready. She didn't answer. I called a few more times with the same results. *No big deal*, I thought. She knew we were coming to get her, so maybe she was in the shower. Or maybe she didn't hear the phone. I kept telling myself I didn't really have any reason to be too concerned. Still, I couldn't shake the feeling that something was wrong.

When Kevin and I arrived at Mom's, I knocked on her front door and she didn't answer. My heart skipped a beat when I saw her car in the driveway. Panic slowly built in me as I dug through my purse frantically searching for the spare key she'd given me to her house. Once we got into the house, Mom was nowhere to be found.

"Mom!" I yelled, running from room to room.

She didn't answer. By then, I was in a full-blown panic. We finally found her at the bottom of the basement stairs. She'd tripped, fallen down the stairs, and couldn't get back up. Fortunately, she'd only sprained her knee, but it could've been much worse.

Although I'd promised Mom I would respect her desire to live alone in the house she'd shared with my dad, seeing her lying helpless at the bottom of the stairs was all I needed to convince myself to break that promise. Mom needed people looking out for her. She needed her family. That day, Mom came to live with us permanently.

Our house wasn't huge, and truth be told, we'd begun to outgrow it. Still, the space was manageable for a family of six. When Mom moved in, our small home suddenly felt very cramped, and we had to make some changes. My oldest son, Mike, who was fifteen at the time, graciously sacrificed his room for Mom and slept on an air mattress in the laundry room for the next two years. His concession made our home livable for everyone, and we were happy in that tiny, shared space for a while, but eventually it became evident we needed a bigger home.

In 2000, we built a much larger home with two extra bedrooms that allowed us to live much more comfortably than before. Mike got his personal space back, and Mom had a room on the main level of the two-story house. That main-level bedroom for Mom eased a good deal of stress because we didn't have to worry about her falling down the stairs. As long as she stayed on the first floor, she was safe. We also had the builder add three-foot-wide doors to Mom's room and bathroom. Making these doorways slightly bigger made it much easier for ambulance stretchers and wheelchairs to move in and out of the room.

In Chinese culture, there's something called *Xiao*, or filial piety. It's a layered concept that's rooted in the strict belief that children have a duty to their parents to care for them in old age. This responsibility usually falls to the oldest son, but my brother Ning wasn't in a position to care for Mom, not like I could. So, I assumed the responsibility. Not only did I bring her into my family's home and gave her a safe environment to live in, Kevin and I also helped her financially, paying her cell phone bill and car insurance.

Was it easy? Not at all. Mom and I had a contentious relationship throughout my formative years, and I still held some bitterness in my heart toward how she handled the situation with my dad, but I tried my best to put all that aside. My siblings weren't available or able to help. The responsibility fell to me. Although I was the youngest, I had a solid financial foundation and the home life to take care of Mom best—and it felt like the right thing to do. Still, I had mixed feelings because it wasn't my responsibility to take care of Mom, not according to Chinese custom. It should've been my oldest brothers' responsibilities, but that's not how it played out. Also, as time went on, it would become more and more difficult to care for Mom physically, emotionally, and financially, but we'll get to that later. But in the early 2000s, it was manageable—and then our family grew.

In August of 2004, Kevin and I welcomed our son, Kaden, and our daughter, Kameyrn, into this world. Holding my twins, one in each arm, was life-affirming and utterly frightening. I loved my babies so much, but it had been nearly two decades since I'd held a newborn in my arms, and I had not one newborn depending on me but two. I had built a great life for myself and our family, but those early days of new motherhood were brutal. I had severe postpartum depression, something I hadn't experienced after my previous four pregnancies. I loved my twins more than life itself and had gone through several rounds of IVF and an emotionally wrecking miscarriage with triplets to get to be their mom. But my postpartum depression didn't allow me to care for them the way I wanted and needed to. Fortunately, my mom stepped in, comforting me and reassuring me when I needed her the most. Her protective love was grander and more visible than when I was a child. I'd never felt that from her before. I craved it and rejected it. Could I believe Mom had really changed?

Something that was different with the twins from when I had my older children was Mom's presence in their lives. Mom no longer worked, and her living with us gave her the opportunity to form a special bond with Kaden and Kameryn. A smile always finds its way to my face when I remember the way her eyes lit up whenever she was with them. Those two precious babies were her pride and joy. She'd do anything for them. As they got older, she'd take them to lunch or to the toy store, letting each pick out a special toy. When the twins started preschool, Mom dropped them off and picked them up. Not only was that special for her, but it helped me out enormously. I finally had some breathing room and didn't feel pulled in a million directions.

And then one day the twins' preschool called. Mom hadn't picked them up. I tried not to panic, but my heart fell to my feet. Mom had been picking up the twins every day for over a year. I didn't call her to learn what happened. I just stopped what I was doing and raced to the school to get Kaden and Kameryn, the whole while thinking, *What's going on with Mom?*

Her forgetting to get the twins wasn't usual. Like I said, she'd been doing it for a long time, but there'd been some incidents, especially with the twins, leading up to this moment that had been concerning to me—or at least raised my antenna. Off and on, Mom would get lost on the way home from her daily trips with them. When they were gone for a long time and finally got home, Mom's reason was, "Oh, I got lost. I couldn't remember how to get home." She'd laugh and shrug it off. To her, it wasn't a big deal. So, we laughed it off too. Her flippant response gave us a false sense of security. If Mom didn't think it was a problem, why should we? After all, she would know if there was something to worry about. Right?

Mom probably had an idea something was off, but like many people in the early stages of dementia, they don't recognize what's happening. They have little insight into their unusual behaviors. Slight deviations from their daily patterns seem like nothing more than a lapse in judgment, tiredness, or plain forgetfulness. A good deal of dementia and Alzheimer's patients and their families chalk up these behaviors to getting older. My family was no different.

After picking up the twins from school, we returned home and found Mom asleep in her bed. Her not picking up the twins was upsetting, but again, I shrugged it off. Everyone's forgotten to set an alarm once in a while. People oversleep. Mom didn't make a habit of doing this. It was the first time, so while I was concerned, I still didn't think it was a problem. I hadn't seen that this incident was a sign, a billboard with flashing neon lights, begging me to pay attention that something was wrong—not just in that moment, but to all the other moments leading up to it.

5

This Food Is Not Rotten

Mom loved to cook and knew her way around the kitchen. Some of her favorite meals to cook were beef broccoli, beef with green beans, chicken and noodles, and soups. The tantalizing aroma of herbs and spices made your mouth water, and we all looked forward to the dishes she prepared until she started cooking rotten food. What used to be a pleasant odor wafting from the kitchen became an awful stench that permeated the entire house.

"Mom, did you cook rotten meat?" I asked one day.

"Why would I cook rotten food?" she answered indignantly.

"It's okay. I haven't cleaned out the fridge lately. It was just a mistake," I said, trying not to make her angry.

Mom had always been a moody person, prone to agitation and disagreeableness, but she'd become more easily annoyed and quick to anger lately. When she first came to live with us, I explained away her increasing mood swings on getting used to a new environment and living in a house full of unique personalities. However, as time went on, the moodiness only worsened.

"How about we order pizza tonight?" I suggested.

My suggestion didn't sit well with Mom, who felt offended that I didn't want to eat the meal she'd spent time making.

"This food is not rotten, Bing," she insisted. Her voice started to rise.

"I'm not trying to hurt your feelings, Mom, but this food has expired. It's definitely rotten."

"Fine!" she yelled. "Then don't eat my cooking." No matter how much I tried to assure her the problem wasn't her cooking, just the spoiled ingredients she used, she felt insulted and lashed out at me. She believed I didn't appreciate her cooking, which was her contribution to the family.

Cooking rotten food wasn't the only problem Mom started exhibiting in the kitchen. Sometimes, she would boil water and leave it on the stove so long it completely evaporated. Once or twice, we'd find her searching the kitchen frantically, looking for food she insisted she'd cooked for us. When we told her she hadn't cooked anything, she thought we were tricking her. Then there were the times when she would start cooking something, forget she'd been cooking, and walk away from the stove, leaving the food to burn on the stove. These incidents were frightening and left me wondering what was happening to her. I can't tell you how many nightmares I had about her accidentally poisoning the kids with rancid meat or burning the house down.

Before the cooking incidents, I noticed another change in Mom. She had trouble remembering how to spell simple words or say certain things in English. Her first language was Cantonese, so it was easy for me to shrug off the minor lapses in her memory as senior moments. *Mom's just getting older,* I'd tell myself. Everyone gets more forgetful with age, and I told myself she wasn't any different. Forgetting words happens from time to time. I'd even been guilty of forgetting a word or phrase now and again. It's common at any age to have moments when we struggle to find words for what we mean to say. And since Cantonese was her first language, it was much easier to ignore what hindsight would later clearly reveal: Mom was slowly forgetting English.

Families miss the signs of early Alzheimer's and dementia all the time because the changes in their loved ones happen gradually. The changes we do recognize like increased forgetfulness, getting lost, and having trouble communicating and mispronouncing words, we explain away as part of the normal aging process, especially since most people begin exhibiting early symptoms of Alzheimer's and dementia in their 60s, 70s, and 80s. According to an Alzheimer's Society survey, "One in three people (33%) who notice symptoms of dementia in themselves or a loved one keep their fears to themselves for over a month." As many as twenty-three percent of loved ones and affected individuals stay quiet for as many as six months before they seek medical help. It's difficult to differentiate when normal memory loss becomes something much more.

Actor Bruce Willis, known for his performances in *Moonlighting*, the *Die Hard* movies, and *Pulp Fiction*, was diagnosed with aphasia and frontotemporal dementia in 2022. Although not Alzheimer's, some of his symptoms mimic those of Alzheimer's patients, and like my experience with Mom,

Willis's daughter and caregiver, Tallulah Willis, didn't think too much of his personality changes right away. She told Rob Haskell in a May 2023 *Vogue* article that although the early signs of her father's cognitive decline were clear in hindsight, at the time, she passed them off as "Hollywood hearing loss" or "vague unresponsiveness." She also admits to taking those early unbeknownst-to-her symptoms personally.

It's hard not to. When Mom called me a thief and liar and accused me of stealing her credit card information, it felt like she'd punched me in the gut. As quarrelsome as she could get with me, she'd never crossed the line of making such absurd allegations. After all I'd done to support and care for her, why would she make such horrible accusations? It was out of character for her.

Still, my focus wasn't entirely on figuring out why Mom thought I'd do something like that. Instead, I had a serious situation that needed to get fixed: getting to the bottom of why Mom's credit card balances were so high.

I called the credit card companies and discovered no one had stolen Mom's card information. Instead, she'd signed up for multiple credit protection programs. The card companies had solicited these programs to Mom, offering her free trials. She'd forgotten she'd signed up for the programs and never canceled the memberships after the free trial expired. Finding out this information didn't surprise me. Mom never understood English well when people talked to her quickly. With her English-language skills declining, any time telemarketers called, Mom handed off the call to me to speak with them. The problem with this strategy is when I wasn't available, she would say yes to anything they offered. I assumed that her confusion and hearing the word "free" led her to say yes to what she thought was a forever no-cost program, not a free trial.

The free credit protection trials weren't the only programs Mom had signed up for. The other charges on her credit cards were from a books-by-mail company. This particular program sent books to readers to read for thirty days. After the thirty-day period ended, the books-by-mail company would charge the credit card on file. I had no idea Mom had been receiving these books. I was the primary income earner of the household, which meant I worked long hours every day and often didn't get home until Mom was asleep. I had no idea the postal service had been delivering books to her, but the evidence was in her room.

Here's what you need to know about Mom: She spent most of her time hidden away in her bedroom, and it was a cluttered mess. For as long as I could remember, she'd been somewhat of a hoarder, although if Mom were reading this book, she'd probably prefer me to call her a collector. She was also very protective of her private space. If myself, Kevin, or the kids went into her room, she'd reprimand them for touching her belongings when all they wanted to do was talk to her. So no one went into Mom's room regularly, which is why no one knew anything was out of the ordinary.

After speaking with the credit card companies, I searched Mom's room for the books and found many of them in unopened boxes piled up alongside other junk items. We spent months returning all those books, but eventually we managed to return them and the charges were credited back to her credit cards.

Mom didn't have many bills since we handled most of those obligations for her. However, money management is often an issue for people with AD. In the early stages of a dementia-related disease, individuals usually have no problems paying bills, but they often have difficulty with more complex tasks like budgeting and can forget that they've taken money out of their bank accounts or authorized charges on their credit cards. Another common sign of dementia-related money management problems is unusual new merchandise purchases showing up in one's home, like Mom's unopened book packages.

Looking back, I probably should've put Mom's credit cards in a safe place where she couldn't find them, but you only know what you know at the moment. But after getting the credit card debacle straightened out and sharing the information with my siblings, one thing was very clear. Something was wrong with Mom. We decided it was time to have her tested for dementia.

6

The Unraveling String of Hope

The thought of Mom not being Mom wasn't something I was ready to accept even though it was clear she was slowly beginning to change. She had many of the textbook traits associated with dementia: confusion, memory loss, mood changes, and impaired judgment. Still, even while sitting at the doctor's office with her, I kept hoping I was overreacting and she'd pass her tests with flying colors, and I could stop worrying that she had a progressive illness.

Testing for Alzheimer's and other forms of dementia, including vascular, frontotemporal, and dementia with Lewy bodies (the kind the late actor Robin Williams had), varies from doctor to doctor, and not one singular test can diagnose if a person is living with any form of dementia. Most doctors rely on a variety of diagnostic tools to make a "probable" or "possible" diagnosis. They make an educated determination based on the patient's medical history; brain imaging results from MRIs, CTs, and PETs; blood tests; cerebrospinal fluid draws; and neurological exams and cognitive and functional assessments, such as being shown a series of words and repeating them after a short time lapse. Even with all these diagnostic tools at their disposal, it's impossible to one hundred percent provide a patient with an Alzheimer's diagnosis until after the individual has passed and their brain tissue can be examined.

Mom's first round of tests were inconclusive and her doctor placed her in the possible category for AD. A possible AD diagnosis means the patient's behaviors aren't typical of AD, but no other cause for the behaviors is known or found. The lack of decisive findings gave me some hope that Mom didn't have any form of dementia, especially Alzheimer's. The possible AD diagnosis strengthened my belief that Mom was just forgetful and acting like a perfectly normal woman in her late 60s, even though she cooked rotten food and forgot about the charges she made to her credit cards. If the doctors weren't sure she had AD, then I felt justified continuing to hold onto the hope that she didn't have it either.

Mom, on the other hand, probably knew her brain was failing her long before we were ready to accept it. The supporting evidence was she became sneakier about hiding her forgetfulness. If someone asked her a question she should know the answer to but didn't, she'd turn the question around on them. For example, if you asked her what day it was, she didn't skip a beat. She'd smile, wave off the question, and say, "You tell me what day it is." She might have struggled to know if it was a Wednesday or a Saturday, but her mind was still sharp enough to hide her memory loss. That's the dementia paradox, and it's why so many people struggle to feel confident in their beliefs that something is wrong with their loved ones.

What I learned from my experience with AD and Mom's

journey is that it's not a linear one. Some days everything seems perfectly normal and other days take you completely by surprise, reminding you that you can't let your guard down with AD.

***

"Bing, Kevin is sneaking into my room. He is writing on my walls in Cantonese," Mom told me one morning before I left for work.

"Mom, Kevin isn't writing on your walls. Maybe you're mistaking the paint pattern for words."

"No, I'm not. I know what I'm seeing, Bing. Someone's written on my walls, and it's Kevin."

"He doesn't even know Chinese. How could it be him?"

"I know it's Kevin. Who else could it be?"

Mom refused to listen to reason. No one and nothing could convince her that her walls weren't covered in writing, so she started locking her door more to keep everyone out of her room.

I learned to live with most of Mom's odd accusations and minor memory lapses. Without a probable AD diagnosis, I still held onto a string of hope, albeit an unraveling string, that what we were seeing with Mom was nothing more than normal aging. Denial is so common for loved ones of an Alzheimer's or dementia patient. You try to convince yourself that the person you love so dearly hasn't changed. You try to normalize their behaviors. Every day you hope they'll get better, and some days they are. Some days are quite calm and event-free—and then the storm arrives.

It was December 2009. Kevin and I were leaving for a work holiday party when we couldn't find Kaden. I searched the upstairs bedrooms, while Kevin looked for him on the main level and basement. While we were searching for Kaden, we realized Mom was also absent. Kevin checked the garage and discovered Mom's car missing. We figured she'd taken Kaden somewhere and didn't tell us. It wasn't too alarming to find them gone. She would often take one or both of the twins somewhere, but she'd usually tell us. This was the first time she disappeared with one of the kids without telling anyone. What was even stranger was she was supposed to watch the twins while we were at the party. Why would she leave with only Kaden?

"Do you know where Paw Paw and Kaden went?" I asked Kameryn. Paw Paw (although written as "Popo" in Cantonese, our family preferred Paw Paw) is the word for grandmother.

"They went to the toy store," she said.

We were perplexed but not necessarily concerned. Our oldest daughter, Lauren, agreed to stay home with Kameryn so we wouldn't be late to the party. We'd only been at the party for about thirty minutes before Lauren's boyfriend called us. He said the police had come to our home and said Mom and Kaden had been taken to the hospital. They'd gotten our address from Mom's driver's license. That was all the information the officer gave Lauren's boyfriend. There was no information about her or Kaden's health status.

We left the party immediately, not bothering to say goodbyes. What had happened to my mom and my son? My heart was pounding out of my chest as we raced down the highway to the hospital. I was an emotional wreck for the entire drive. My stomach was in knots as I thought about them lying in the hospital. I feared they were seriously injured, or worse, because if everything was fine, Mom would have called me and let me know what had happened. The fear in Kevin's eyes and his white-knuckling of the steering wheel told me he was thinking the same thing. I prayed fiercely to God during that drive, begging and bargaining for their safety. The drive normally would have taken as much as forty minutes, but we made it in twenty.

Once we got to the hospital, we found out neither was seriously injured. In fact, Kaden was perfectly fine and very excited to recount his exciting ride in the ambulance and show us the treats the nurses had given him. We learned Mom had taken Kaden to the toy store like Kameryn told us. She'd fainted while shopping, and the store employees called 911.

The doctors couldn't find anything wrong with Mom, and she had no memory of passing out. She didn't understand why she was at the hospital and wanted to go home immediately. The doctors determined dehydration caused her to faint. They hooked her up to an IV to rehydrate her. While the IV fluids did their work, the doctors ran several more tests on Mom to figure out what else might have caused the fainting episode. Like usual, the tests were inconclusive. The doctor on duty asked us questions about Mom's memory. I told him she'd been forgetting to take her medication, which I knew wasn't good for her because of her diabetes and her eating habits were poor. Sometimes she'd forget to eat. My stomach clenched and the string of hope unraveled even more. I knew where this was going.

He did a few more neurological and cognitive assessments designed specifically to detect AD and dementia. One of the tests was to draw a clock face with a specific time on it and provide the current date. Mom failed this test miserably. By the end of this hospital trip, we were told Mom's possible AD diagnosis had advanced into the probable category.

Obviously this doctor is wrong. That is what I thought when he spoke those words. I didn't believe it one bit. More precisely, I didn't want to believe it. Mom didn't have Alzheimer's. I started playing back scenes from the last few years and all the things that had happened more recently: the credit card charges, the rotten food, her forgetting her way home from the store, forgetting to pick up the kids from school, and not telling us she was leaving with Kaden. Deep down, I always knew something wasn't right, but when you love someone, you don't want to accept that something is seriously wrong. You want them to be healthy because what happens if they're not? What does that future look like?

I had a lot of preconceived ideas of what Alzheimer's looked like. Although I'd known something was wrong with Mom, being handed an AD diagnosis from this doctor felt like the rug being pulled out from under me. Would Mom die soon?

My oldest daughter, Lauren, who is a certified nurse assistant (CNA), had been working at a local skilled nursing facility in the memory care unit when Mom was diagnosed. While I thought the world was ending, Lauren gently explained that Mom wasn't near the end.

"She's fine, Mom."

Fine? How could an AD diagnosis be fine? At that time, I didn't understand the stages of the disease. I thought if you had it, then that's it. You die soon. Lauren patiently told me that's not how AD works.

"Paw Paw is still fairly cognitive. She might be forgetful and have some judgment lapses, but she's okay right now."

I had to believe her, right? What other choice did I have? Of course, I'm not someone who doesn't do her research. I knew I had to be Mom's advocate and make sure she got the best care possible. I just didn't know at the time what that meant. I also didn't realize how much I'd have to manage my siblings' feelings too.

My brother Wai, who was a doctor, already suspected Mom had dementia. So the diagnosis came as no surprise to him. He took the news very matter-of-factly, or maybe clinically is the better word. His training told him everything he needed to know about the situation, and his black-and-white way of thinking about things didn't leave much room for interpretation. He saw

AD as a predetermined path with only one outcome that he had no choice but to accept.

My oldest brother, Ning, was riding the denial roller coaster like me, although maybe more so because he truly believed Mom would be fine once she went home with me. "With the right medication, the right place, everything will get better," he said more than once. His hope and expectations that all would be fine with Mom were completely opposite of Wai's more realistic, and sometimes harsh, approach to Mom's situation. I wanted so badly to buy into Ning's vision that she would recover from what he thought was a minor setback.

Mon's feelings were slightly more complicated. My grandmother and a nanny raised Mon in Hong Kong during the first five years of her life. She'd never really known our parents until they came to Hong Kong for our grandmother's funeral. Mon lived with our parents for about thirteen years, but with her younger years being with relatives in Hong Kong, she never bonded with them or had a deeply loving relationship with Mom. So, while she was sad and had some initial denial like me and Ning, her feelings about the situation were slightly more detached.

My emotions about the AD diagnosis were all over the place. All my life, I sought Mom's approval and never really got it. Some of it had to do with her upbringing and Chinese culture's emphasis on male success. She always gave my brothers' achievements more attention than my own and even gave my sons' achievements more attention than my daughters'. I earned my degrees and worked as hard as I did to provide for my family, but that didn't mean I still didn't want to hear her tell me what a good mother I was or how I'd overcome so much and she was proud of me. With Mom's AD diagnosis, I had to accept I'd probably never get any of that from her.

I knew AD meant Mom would continue to become forgetful, but I didn't understand how it would change her brain. When I heard of people being diagnosed with AD prior to my mom's diagnosis, I thought of senility. I thought it was merely forgetting what day it was or where you put your keys. As I started to learn more about the disease, I learned someday Mom would forget how to eat, how to take a shower, or how to use the toilet. I didn't realize that she might have hallucinations she thought were so real that she'd be left terrified, and I'd be helpless to ease her fears. I had no clue how much this disease would change her personality and her perceptions of reality.

I didn't realize how much it would change my life, too.

7

What Do You Mean I Can't Drive?

Put her in a nursing home. That's what so many well-meaning friends and family members said to me when learning about Mom's diagnosis. "It'll be too hard on you," a good friend told me.

Another friend tried a different approach. "You're so busy, Bing. How will you have time to take care of her?"

While I appreciated their wanting to make things easier for me, they were unfamiliar with the situation. Putting my mom in a nursing home wasn't even a question for me. I'm not saying there's anything wrong with going that route. Sometimes, it's the better option, and families have to do what's right for them and their loved ones. But I knew finding a nursing home that could bridge the language barrier would be tough, if not impossible. Mom had already lost so much of her English-speaking skills because of the disease, and I knew those skills would continue to diminish. She needed to be with people who she could communicate with and who could understand her. Most importantly, I knew she had to have her family around her. In Chinese culture, taking care of one's elders was expected. It should've been the eldest son, but it fell to me because I had the resources and the perceived availability. Also, I wanted to do it.

I knew being a caregiver wouldn't be easy. It would be downright difficult, but I didn't feel there was any other reasonable choice for our situation. Also, aside from the language barrier, how could I not take care of the woman who'd raised me and did her best to care for me? For me, choosing the nursing home route meant putting her in a facility to die—and die faster. Most people sixty-five years and older diagnosed with AD, according to the Alzheimer's Association, die within four to eight years of their initial diagnosis. Some live for as long as twenty years. A few years into Mom's AD, her doctors told me to be ready to let her die because she was getting sick more often. I wasn't ready for her to die. I did my best to fight for her healthcare. She couldn't advocate for herself, so I took on the fight for her. I felt the doctors wrote her off because she was an AD patient. Although they never said these words to me, I felt they didn't want to fight for her because they knew the outcome of AD. Why prolong the inevitable? But Mom lived with that inevitable outcome hanging over her head for sixteen years before she lost her battle with AD. This was ten years after her doctors told me to let her go. I attribute much of those added years to living at home with family and having someone advocate for her. Advocating for Mom wasn't easy because doctors tended to write us off because, once again, of the inevitable outcome, but I had to do it. If I didn't, who would?

Caring for AD patients at home isn't rare either. Whether it's a cultural preference or because finances make it difficult to pay for the cost of memory care, as of the writing of this book, more than eleven million loved ones provide unpaid care for individuals with AD or other dementia types.

It would be an oversight not to include that part of what motivated my desire to care for Mom at home was others' doubt. It fed my desire to care for Mom and prove them wrong. *I could do it.* I could handle the stress of caregiving. When people told me that Mom would forget who I was someday, I wanted to prove them wrong so badly. I refused to accept that caring for her would be too stressful or that it wouldn't matter anyway because she wouldn't know what was happening to appreciate my caregiving. I refused to accept those outcomes.

I might have spent time riding denial's roller coaster, but I knew there were some unavoidable truths to Mom's illness. Like my brother Wai, I knew the final outcome of AD. I knew Mom wouldn't recover from this illness. I knew there wasn't a vaccine or miracle medical treatment that would cure her. It would continue to steal her essence until her last breath. She would die from this dreadful disease. Still, I couldn't stand by idly and wait for her to deteriorate and die.

I did some research and learned that AD patients who were placed in a nursing home had more rapid cognitive decline than those who stayed at home. Being in a familiar environment, surrounded by familiar faces and their belongings, proved highly beneficial. Home-based care also makes it easier for AD patients to participate in their care for as long as possible. The comforts of home and having familiar caregivers nearby is less confusing and scary for the individual, especially as the disease progresses.

Alzheimer's Research and Therapy has determined chronic stress increases not only the risk of developing AD, but speeds up the progression of the disease. Learning all this made it clear to me that keeping Mom at home was the key to maintaining her health and her brain function for longer. I wasn't one hundred percent sure my plan to keep her home until the end would work. We were at the beginning of what I was beginning to understand would be a long, slow journey. Maybe a memory care facility would be better for Mom later on, but at the moment, I couldn't fathom sending her to a nursing home. I felt confident I could care for her best, and the first order of business with my new role as caregiver was delivering news she didn't want to hear.

***

"What do you mean I can't drive?"

Mom was furious when I told her she couldn't drive anymore. After the doctors handed out the AD diagnosis, they recommended we no longer allow Mom to drive. That was a blow to all of us. How do you tell your parent they can no longer drive and take away their freedom and independence?

"Mom, it's too risky. What if you get lost?"

"My memory is fine," she argued. "I don't forget things."

Arguing with her was exhausting. It didn't help the situation if I pointed out she'd already gotten lost before on her trips with the twins or that the day after she came home from the hospital she'd asked Kevin to get her purse from Ning's truck, convinced he'd driven her home.

"Mom," Kevin told her, "Ning didn't bring you home. I brought you home in the van." The only way to placate Mom's insistence was to take her out to Ning's truck and let her look for her purse. Of course she didn't find it.

Every day was a struggle. She couldn't understand why she couldn't drive herself anymore—that she could get lost or hurt or, God forbid, hurt someone else. I tried my best to hold my ground, but it was hard. Taking her keys away not only stole her independence, but it meant more things added to my plate. She'd been picking up the twins from preschool since they started, and I couldn't let her do that anymore.

Still, if you have someone in your life with AD, you know how easy it is to convince yourself that the disease isn't real. Or it's not as bad as everyone says it is. That's why I relented. Like a teenager, Mom did her best to convince me she could still drive. She wasn't a danger to herself or others, she insisted—and so she persuaded me to let her go on short trips. I didn't want her to drive, but I also wanted to believe she was getting better. She was so adamant and confident. Her memory even seemed to improve. She wasn't forgetting things as often, so I convinced myself letting her go on short trips wouldn't be a problem. And for a while it wasn't. She always made it back home without incident.

Then it happened again.

I was in New York City on a business trip when my son, Anthony, called me.

"Mom, Paw Paw Wants to take Kameryn to the store. Is that

okay?"

Was I one hundred percent comfortable with Mom driving my daughter? No, I can't say I was, but she'd been doing so well on her little driving trips that I told myself it would be fine. Honestly, I wasn't sure it would be, but that's what makes the role of caregiving for your parent so difficult. You have to set boundaries for the person who used to set them for you. You get a front row seat to watching your parent regress from adulthood to childhood. They change from the independent person you've always known to a scared, angry kid who doesn't understand what's happening to them. They turn into an adult who doesn't remember how to drive a car or how to get home after they've run an errand. The person who taught you how to tie your shoes, how to use the toilet, and how to do all the adult things you do doesn't remember how to do those things for themselves. They become dependent on you, and they hate it because they don't understand. And, to be completely honest, you hate it too at times. You might feel love and compassion for your AD parent, but that doesn't mean you aren't upset about your role as their caregiver and the freedom you've given up to take on that role. You're forced to accept that sometimes life doesn't progress the way you thought. That becoming older doesn't mean becoming wiser. Old age for an AD patient means regressing to infanthood, and it's unsettling.

When Anthony told me Mom wanted to take my youngest daughter to the store, I didn't know what else to say except, "Well, you can't stop her."

I wish I hadn't spoken those words.

***

How many hours was it after I told Anthony we couldn't stop Mom? I don't remember. All I remember is getting a worrisome call from the St. Charles County Fire Department, a call I'd hoped wouldn't come but, if I'm being honest, wasn't surprised to have received.

"Ms. Dempewolf?" The man on the other end asked.

"Yes," I replied hesitantly. It was one of those moments when words catch in your throat because you don't want to speak out of fear of what comes next.

"We've taken your mom to the hospital. She fell at the dollar store. Your daughter is with her."

I hung up the phone and called Kevin. He was on his way to a job interview but didn't hesitate to turn around immediately and go to the hospital to see what was happening. There I was, nearly a thousand miles away from home, and my mom was being taken to the hospital and one of my children was taken with her — again. Is this what my friends tried to warn me about? I knew I wore stubborn glasses and refused to believe caring for Mom and managing my career wouldn't be as bad as everyone thought, but had they seen things more clearly from the get-go? Had they told me something like this would happen and I'd be sitting alone and helpless in New York waiting for news, would it have changed my mind? Perhaps it might have given me pause, but I can't say it would've changed my mind. As the minutes and hours ticked by while I waited to hear from Kevin, it was an excruciating waiting game. All I wanted was to be by her side. My stomach was in knots, and I blamed myself for what happened. I should've told Anthony to stop Mom.

When Kevin finally called, the news wasn't good. Mom had broken her left hip, her left elbow, and would need surgery. I couldn't be by Mom's side for the surgery, but I could get her the best treatment possible.

"Call Timothy," I told Kevin. Timothy was a family friend and an orthopedic surgeon. If there was anyone I trusted to do Mom's surgery, it was him.

Kevin made the call, and Mom was transferred to a different hospital in St. Charles for her surgery the next day. I was still in New York and was trying my best to get back as quickly as possible, but I couldn't find a last-minute flight for less than a thousand dollars. I was left with no other choice but to stay in New York, so I called Wai and asked him to be with Kevin while Mom was in surgery. Mom needed her family there, and while Kevin's presence was soothing, she needed her children by her side. Wai made the two-hour drive from Cape Girardeau in Missouri's Bootheel to St. Charles.

When I finally made it home, Mom's mental state was worse than ever before. The surgery had gone well, but she couldn't remember what had happened to land her in the hospital.

"Bing, my elbow hurts," she cried.

"I know it does, Mom. It's because you had surgery."

She shook her head at me and became even more distressed. "No. No. No, I didn't have surgery."

To say it was heartbreaking to see her so confused and in such distress, unaware of why she was in the hospital again, is an understatement. If you're reading this book and caring for a loved one at this stage in their AD journey, you know "heartbreaking" isn't a strong enough term to do the painful feelings justice.

Mom stayed in the hospital for five days, followed by six weeks at a nursing home for rehab. Yes, the irony wasn't lost on me. I'd been so adamant she'd never step foot in a nursing home, and yet, there she was. And of course, I blamed myself. That's a symptom of caregiving no one tells you about: how much blame you take and how it feels like taking a million punches to the gut repeatedly. One positive aspect of Mom being in the nursing home was that my daughter Lauren worked there as a CNA. Although she couldn't care for her directly because she was family, it was reassuring to know that she could check on her if needed.

Mom was equally upset about her current living situation. She was fiercely opposed to being moved to the rehab center at the nursing home, telling anyone who would listen that she wasn't told about the move and didn't consent to it. I tried to reassure her that she was in good hands. I wanted to believe that was true, but I'd heard stories about how nursing facilities mistreated their patients, leaving them sitting for hours unattended, neglected, and even abused. I desperately wanted to believe these were over-the-top stories that weren't the norm. After all, I had no other choice at that point but to give in and trust that Mom would get the care she needed while she recovered.

It took less than an hour upon Mom's admittance to the rehab facility before things began to break down.

8

The Blame Game

"I have to go to the bathroom," Mom told me after they wheeled her into her room and left.

"Okay," I said. "Let me get someone to help."

I pressed the nurse call button and we waited. No one came.

"I really have to go," Mom insisted like a child.

Not wanting her to soil herself, I helped her to the bathroom. Thirty minutes later, someone finally responded to our call.

"Why did you take her to the bathroom?" the nursing home staff member asked quite rudely.

"She had to go and no one came to help."

"Well, in the future, all bathroom trips can only be handled by a staff member."

I stared at the staff member incredulously. Was she joking? I couldn't help my mom to the bathroom? When I questioned her, she explained that it was a liability issue for anyone other than staff to move patients. I understood the liability concern, but what baffled me was the slowness of the staff's response. It seemed they didn't care. It took too long to get a response. What if Mom had fallen and needed help getting up? Worse, what if she'd fallen and gotten hurt, worsening the injuries she was there to recover from? They had no idea why we rang the nurse call button. It could've been for any number of reasons. Yes, I understood there were other patients the staff was caring for, but thirty minutes? That was too long of a response time for me to accept, and that's when I decided Mom would never be left alone in the rehab facility for any longer than necessary if I could help it, even if it meant my days suddenly got longer.

I got to the nursing home every morning by six o'clock to help with her morning routine. By eight o'clock, I had to leave to begin my workday. That's when a private caregiver we hired, Sharon, relieved me. She stayed with Mom throughout the day so she wouldn't be alone until I could make it back. Most days, I finished work between five and six in the evening and then headed back to the nursing facility where I'd stay until eight or nine o'clock before heading home thoroughly exhausted. So many times during those weeks driving home at night, my eyes felt heavy. I'm so grateful I never fell asleep at the wheel.

My weekends were also spent by Mom's side. I'd spend Saturdays and Sundays with her from six or seven in the morning until nine or ten at night. During this time, Kevin held down the fort at home, taking care of Kaden and Kameryn, who were five, making dinner for the family, and basically running the household alone. To this day, I don't know how I would've managed this schedule without his help.

Some people might have believed my reaction was excessive. *Really, Bing*, I imagined them saying to me. *All this because it took the staff a bit of time to respond?* I didn't care if people found it excessive. Was it easy? Absolutely not. But my mom needed me, so I did what was necessary. The first time I deviated from my usual routine, one of my fears came true.

* * *

It was May 9, 2010. Mother's Day. The day before I'd spent my usual time at the nursing facility with Mom. That night when I returned home, I was more exhausted than usual. The grueling schedule started to catch up to me. I knew I needed to rest. My body needed more sleep. I couldn't keep going at the pace I was going. I wasn't ready to give up my caregiving schedule, but certainly I could sleep in a little the next day. It would be a Mother's Day gift to myself.

When I arrived at the nursing facility later in the day to see Mom, she had two bruises on her arm that I one hundred percent knew weren't there the night before. One was a half-dollar size bruise on the outer part of her arm. The second bruise was on the underside of her arm and much larger. It was nearly four inches long and an inch wide. I know that as we age, we bruise more easily. The skin becomes thinner and the blood vessels are protected less from injury because the protective fatty layer that acts as a cushion loses some of its plumpness. But those weren't bruises from accidentally hitting oneself on a bed rail.

What was worse? No one at the nursing facility could tell me where they came from. The only response to Mom's mysterious bruises was from a supervisor who told me they'd have to open an investigation to figure out what led to the bruising. To this day, I believe that was a line to pacify me, not reassure me. I don't believe for one moment an investigation was opened because, after that day, I never heard anything else about the incident. I didn't have the answers I sought, and my heart wept for my mom.

And, once again, I blamed myself. I'd been so careful making sure Sharon or I was with Mom so something like that wouldn't happen. Yet the first moment I deviated from the normal routine, look what happened. I told myself the story that if I'd been there, those bruises and whatever caused them wouldn't have happened. I berated myself for letting Mom down, for letting myself down. Time puts so much in the rearview mirror, helping us see situations clearer than when we're in them at the moment. Looking back, I know that I tasked myself with the impossible job of controlling the situation. I had tried to do everything I could to keep something like that from happening to my mom, but what control did I really have? But attempting to control an uncontrollable situation like caring for a loved one with AD often gives caregivers some semblance of order and purpose.

As upset as I was about the unexplained bruises, the straw that broke the camel's back came two weeks later. A family friend went with me to visit Mom, and when we walked into her room, we found her slumped over in a wheelchair by her bed and the overwhelming scent of urine hit our noses. Mom was soaked in urine, and I had no idea how long she'd sat there like that. As I rushed over to her, my friend hit the nurse call button—and, like the last time, no one came. No way was I going to wait for

God knows how long for someone to come clean her up. I rolled the wheelchair with Mom in it straight into the shower. She didn't like that one bit and fought me, saying she didn't need a shower.

"Mom, you've urinated on yourself," I explained gently. "I just want to help you get cleaned up. You'll feel much better."

"I'm not a baby, Bing. I know how to use the bathroom."

Convincing her of what had happened was futile. Then, as I tried to clean her up, she defecated in the shower. I tried to keep my composure, but standing in the shower, already trying to clean my urine-soaked mother while she defecated on herself, sent me reeling. *What is happening?* I thought. Had she forgotten she was in the shower? She'd been sitting on a shower chair with a hole in the middle, so maybe she was confused and thinking she was on the toilet. Was this the beginning of the downhill slide?

By the time a staff member arrived, I had Mom cleaned up and back in her wheelchair and I was furious. I tried my best to calmly explain that we'd found Mom soaked in urine, slumped in her wheelchair, and that, once again, it had taken at least thirty minutes for someone to respond to our call for help, but my anger was apparent and the staff member could see it.

"There's no way of knowing how long my mom actually sat in her urine," I told the staff member, who didn't have much to say about the incident, which, of course, angered me more. But, honestly, her silence was probably for the best because any explanation or excuse she had given would've made me angrier since I couldn't accept there being any valid reason for taking thirty minutes to respond to a patient's call for help.

I wanted to bring Mom home immediately, but I knew I needed to prepare our home more to take care of Mom better and protect her. For starters, we had to do something about her room. Like I said before, Mom was a hoarder and her room was a nightmare. The piles of junk in her bedroom had to go to ensure her safety. While cleaning, we discovered money and checks hidden in numerous books and magazines written to all sorts of organizations, mostly religious. It appeared Mom had been writing checks to any group that had sent out a request for donations. Thankfully, she never mailed the checks, placing them in between the pages of books and magazines, forgetting about them nearly as quickly as she wrote them. We even found the book of blank checks Mom insisted we had stolen from her. It was a relief to have proof that we weren't stealing from her. Kevin and I knew we hadn't done anything wrong, but it felt good to show my family this proof just to make it very clear that we had never stolen from Mom.

After cleaning up her room, we tackled her bathroom. Like her bedroom, the bathtub had piles of paper in it too, which made it clear to me that she hadn't been bathing as often as she told us she was. I knew sometimes she'd come out of her room and use one of the other showers in the house, but it wasn't often. While removing the papers from the tub, I thought about all the things I'd have to help Mom with when she came home. I would need to remind her to bathe and most likely have to help her. Since she was becoming more and more incontinent, eventually I'd have to change her adult diapers and make sure she stayed clean. The amount of care Mom would need would only continue to increase. I'm not going to lie. I wasn't looking forward to it. The thought of providing the level of care Mom would need for the next who-knows-how-many years felt overwhelming. I knew I needed to get prepared. So, I bought as many books as I could find on caregiving, read as much as I could read online, hell- bent on consuming as much information as possible to make sure I knew what I was doing. Spoiler alert: We never know as much as we think when caring for an AD or dementia patient. We learn the ropes as we go along.

After we emptied Mom's room, we redecorated it, repainting the walls and replacing the carpeting. We installed handrails in the bathroom to reduce her risk of falling and make it easier for her to use the toilet. We even placed a baby monitor in her room so I could hear her if she needed me or something happened. My siblings even helped pay for some of the costs to make Mom's room safe and a peaceful environment. Although the cost to redecorate her room wasn't too expensive, it felt good to know my siblings were willing to contribute.

We, meaning me, Kevin, and my siblings, felt prepared for Mom to return home and for the obstacles that lay ahead. I felt like the preparations I'd completed and the research I'd done had put me ahead of Mom's disease, but that didn't mean I didn't cry myself to sleep most nights. Mom wasn't supposed to be sick. I wasn't supposed to be raising a young family and caring for Mom too. Just when she had come back into my life in a meaningful way, AD stole her from me. I needed her.

Maybe it sounds selfish, but I was angry at God, the Universe, whoever or whatever, because the plans I had for my life had been ripped out from underneath me like the proverbial rug. I wasn't financially independent. I wasn't retired. I was a middle-aged woman working and raising my family. I needed Mom to be there for me like she wasn't when I was younger—and she was, for a while. She'd been someone I could count on to be there for Kaden and Kameryn. She got them on and off the bus. She was with them after school. But with Mom's AD progressing faster than I wanted to admit, she couldn't do that anymore. Instead of her being there for me, I had to be there for her and everyone else. None of us think when we're in the prime of our lives that we'll be taking care of sick parents, but it happens. Children caregiving for parents, multigenerational households, those situations have always existed, but as people live longer and dementia illnesses are on the rise, it's only going to become more of the norm. While I can say that matter-of-factly, to actually live it is another beast entirely. I never thought I'd have to take care of my mom or watch her revert back to childhood, acting like a toddler and fighting with her about eating or bathing. With such a full, busy life already, I didn't know how I'd manage to take care of Mom, but I knew I had to find a way.

9

Curveballs

Bringing Mom home to live with us after my dad died felt right. I felt prepared to care for her. Even after her probable AD diagnosis, I felt confident I could handle her care. This time was completely different. I was an emotional wreck, and self-doubt infused every cell in my body. This time I understood that caring for Mom would continue to get increasingly difficult.

To prepare for Mom's return to our home, in addition to cleaning her room and getting the house ready, I read anything I could find about caring for people diagnosed with AD. I spent hours scouring the Internet, consuming as much information as I could about caregiving and AD. I read *The 36-Hour Day* by Nancy L. Mace and Peter V. Rabins, which would become my bible. As you know, the Internet is a double-edged sword when it comes to information. On one hand, you can find information about anything you want and get connected with people experiencing the same things you are. It's also the scariest rabbit hole to go down. I'd stay up late most nights reading the most terrifying information about what AD does to the person diagnosed with it and those caring for their loved ones. Although I knew on an intellectual level that Mom would forget me, my siblings, my children, and grandchildren, seeing it in black and white on a computer screen in a Facebook group or written in a best-selling book made it more real than I wanted it to be. But like I said, the Internet is a double-edged sword because there was comfort in learning that some of the things Mom had been doing weren't out of spite or punishing me for being a bad daughter. Yes, even though years had passed since my girlhood, I still held a lot of trauma in my mind and body from my mom's seemingly lack of concern toward my dad's abuse. So, when she'd lash out at me or accuse me of stealing, I couldn't help but feel tremors in my bones from her long-ago and not-so-long-ago accusations. Reading others' experiences with their loved ones who'd done the same things made me feel less attacked and more understanding that the abusive tirades and hurtful accusations were the disease acting out, not my mom. She didn't really believe what she said. It was the disease lying to her, making her suspicious that people were trying to harm her and fueling the changes in her personality and temperament, like her violent outbursts and delusional behaviors.

Still, after reading about what the future held for Mom and for me and my family, I started to feel downright terrified of my decision to keep her in our home. It didn't help that friends and family were continuing to tell me that I couldn't be a caregiver, more so now than when Mom first was diagnosed with probable AD. *She has to be in a nursing home. She can't stay at home. You can't take care of her. She'll die soon.* I didn't want to hear those things. I wanted everyone who spoke those defeatist words to be wrong, but as humans, we're sponges. Try as we might, most of us soak up others' opinions and words and start to believe them. I did. I felt overwhelmed by what lay ahead, and I doubted myself nonstop. Could I really be the caregiver that my mom needed? Could I keep her safe in our home? I had a career, six children, eight grandchildren, and a husband. How many more roles could I add to my already busy life?

When the self-doubt was at its worst, Kevin sat me down and said, "Just stop for a second. Your Mom lives with us, not anyone else. With all due respect to them, no one else understands what's going on in our home. You tell me what you want to do, and we'll make it happen."

To this day, I'm not sure Kevin knows what that moment meant to me. I felt heard and empowered, less uncertain and fully supported by the person on this journey with me, my husband. I took a deep breath and answered truthfully.

"I want her home with us."

Kevin took my hands in his and said, "Then we'll keep her home."

My heart overflowed with love for him. He'd been my rock throughout the whole ordeal, and now, he was supporting me unwaveringly in the decision to care for my mom. With Kevin's support, I knew I could care for Mom. It wouldn't be easy, but Kevin's belief gave me strength.

I had no clue what was in store for us beyond the bleak outlook that books and online articles detailed, but I knew one thing for sure: A strong network of love and support is essential when caring for someone with dementia—and I knew, without a doubt, that I had that network with Kevin by my side. We'd weather all the seasons of AD together, and let me tell you, weathering such a beast of a disease isn't something I'd wish on my worst enemy.

* * *

Day-to-day life with Mom, once she came home from the nursing home, was a struggle. We never knew what to expect from her from one moment to the next. She'd have stunning moments of clarity when she seemed to remember everything about her life. Then, a few minutes later, she'd forget what day it was or who she was talking to.

Mom had only been home a few months before she began falling frequently. The first time it happened, Lauren and her boyfriend found her on the floor in her room. When they tried to help her up, she complained her hips hurt and she couldn't put weight on her legs. Lauren called 911 and then she called me. I was in the middle of an interview at a nearby restaurant with a potential candidate for a position at my company.

"Mom, we just found Paw Paw on the floor in her room and —"

Before she could finish speaking, my default panic mode kicked in. I began yelling into the phone.

"What happened? Did you call 911?"

I never let her answer. Instead, I rushed out of the restaurant, nearly forgetting to pay the bill, called my assistant to let her know what was happening, and sped all the way home. By the time I arrived, the paramedics were in my home. They helped Mom get up off the floor and had her seated in a chair at the kitchen table. She managed to get herself in the chair with the assistance of her walker, they told me. When I asked if she needed to go to the hospital, they told me she refused to go.

"She says she's fine," one of the paramedics told me. "We can't force her to go."

This upset me tremendously because I felt Mom needed to get checked out.

"Listen, my mom has dementia. She's probably confused," I tried to explain. Still, the paramedics wouldn't budget.

"If she says she's fine, we can't make her go."

To say I was frustrated is putting it mildly. How could I make them understand how AD made Mom believe things that weren't sensible? Surely, these medical professionals understood dementia diseases and how they worked. But what I'd learned throughout the duration of Mom's illness, especially during the times she was more coherent around strangers who didn't understand AD and its fickleness, was that unless Mom was exhibiting clear signs of confusion and dementia, her wishes trumped mine or any caregivers. As a caregiver, that was one of the hardest things to manage, knowing Mom couldn't make the best decisions for herself and me having no say in those decisions. I wanted Mom to get checked out at the hospital. She didn't want to go, and to the paramedics, there was no middle ground. Mom's wishes took precedence.

Fortunately, in my case, I had power of attorney. I'd gotten it before Mom had completely lost her memory to ensure its validity. I'd merely forgotten this important fact in the midst of pleading with the paramedics. Thank goodness Lauren remembered.

"My mom has power of attorney, and she gets to make the final call," she told the paramedics.

The words "power of attorney" turned the situation on its head immediately. The paramedics wanted my opinion after all, asking me if I wanted her to go to the hospital. While I was so certain that's what was necessary thirty seconds earlier, now that the decision was in my hands, I started to second-guess myself, something caregivers do often. If you're reading this book and you're caring for someone with AD or another form of dementia, know that uncertainty is normal. It's part of the vicious cycle of caring for a person who can't make decisions for themselves.

"I don't know if I want her to go to the hospital. Is anything broken?"

The paramedics told me they didn't think anything was broken and an immediate trip to the hospital probably wasn't necessary.

"Are you in pain, Mom?" I asked in Chinese. "How are you feeling?" Even though I knew I had the final call on whether she went to the hospital, I still wanted to include her in the decision. I wanted her to feel heard and spoken to, not spoken about.

Confusion then irritation spread across her face. "I'm fine,

Bing. Why would I be in pain?"

"You fell, Mom. Remember?"

"I didn't fall."

"But, Mom, Lauren found you lying on the floor."

"I didn't fall. I sat down on the floor."

Mom had either already forgotten she'd fallen or was trying to cover it up. It was always so hard to know what she knew and didn't know. Regardless, I decided she didn't need to go to the emergency room. After the paramedics left, Lauren and I helped her to her bed so she could rest. Next, I called Mom's doctor to let him know what happened and what we should do next. He wasn't surprised she'd fallen or had forgotten what had happened. He told me to bring her into his office the next day to have X-rays taken to make sure nothing was broken. He also used the incident as an opportunity to tell me what so many others had told me: She should be in a nursing home and our house wasn't safe for her.

I hung up the phone, furious at her doctor for telling me I couldn't handle the situation. Tired and stressed from the whole ordeal, I needed someone to take it out on. I turned on Lauren, lashing out at her and accusing her of not caring for Mom well.

"Why weren't you checking on her? How could you let her fall?" I yelled.

"I did check on her, Mom!" she yelled back. "She was perfectly fine. I went to make her lunch and when I went back into her room to tell her lunch was ready, she was on the floor.

It happened that fast. I wasn't ignoring her. I can't be with her every minute."

I might have asked Lauren what happened, but I have to admit that at that moment I didn't want to hear what she had to say. Instead, I stomped out of the house to get back to work and left Lauren to watch Mom. I didn't get too far down the road before regret filled every inch of my body. I felt horrible taking out my stress and fear on my daughter. Lauren had been such a blessing and so helpful with Mom. Once again, I realized the person I was most angry with wasn't her, the clueless paramedics, or her scolding doctor. I was most mad at myself because I wasn't there to stop Mom from falling. I knew Lauren did her best caring for Mom. I knew she wasn't responsible for Mom's accident either, and thankfully, aside from a few minor bruises, Mom was fine.

Caregiving was taking its toll on my mental health. It was straining my relationships with my loved ones. The care strategies I'd put in place would only work for so long because Mom's condition would only worsen with time. I started to realize that my impatience and anger was a sign that I needed more support, but I didn't know how to ask for it. It was difficult enough for me, a high-achieving woman, to juggle my needs while meeting my mom's. How could I ask others to take on the burden? How could I ask my siblings, two of whom lived too far away to offer much physical support, to share the responsibility? To say I felt trapped is an understatement.

A few nights after the falling incident, I heard Mom on the baby monitor around midnight moaning. I bolted out of bed and ran downstairs in my nightgown to check on her. I found her lying face down on the floor next to the bed with her legs in the air against the bed.

"Mom! Mom! Are you okay? What happened?" I asked as I helped her maneuver herself into a sitting position.

"I was getting up to go to the bathroom and slid out of bed. I'm fine."

That was Mom's mantra: "I'm fine." Clearly, she wasn't fine, but I knew arguing with her wouldn't help. So I let it go. I looked her over for signs of broken bones or bleeding. She had carpet burns and swelling on the right side of her face and forehead. That familiar feeling of guilt began creeping into my body again. The little voice in my head said, *You did this. You should've been down there to protect her. Her carpet burns and swollen face are all your fault!*

I couldn't lift Mom myself, so I yelled in the baby monitor to Kevin. He came downstairs quickly and helped me get her back into bed. Like a small child, she rolled to one side, her back to us, and went back to sleep. Kevin put his arm around my shoulders and asked if I was okay.

"I don't know what I am right now," I answered. I felt helpless as well as responsible for Mom falling out of bed. I hugged Kevin and thanked him for his help. Then I sent him back to bed while I got an ice pack for Mom's swollen face.

"Are you sure? I can stay here and help if you need me."

I looked into his eyes and forced a smile. I nodded shortly and kissed his cheek, assuring him I was fine. Hesitantly, he went back to bed, while I went back to Mom's room with the ice pack and lay in bed with her, holding the pack on her face while she slept. As I lay there, my mind raced. *Was everyone right? Did Mom belong in a nursing home or memory care facility?* Those places had night staff, which I didn't have in my home. But could they have even stopped her from falling? I thought about Mom's rehabilitation stay and how we'd found her soaked in urine slumped in the wheelchair. I remembered the bruises I'd found on her on Mother's Day. How long would she have lain on the laminate floor before staff had found her?

Then I thought about my role in this most recent fall. What could I have done differently to prevent it? The baby monitor had been instrumental in finding her quickly after her fall because I heard her moans. But then I had to ask myself a more pointed question: How long would she have laid on the floor in her room if I hadn't had the baby monitor? Maybe I needed video monitors in her room, but that idea made me feel even guiltier. Was it right to have her watched at all times like a caged animal, making her a prisoner in her room? Like many caregivers who want the best for their loved ones, I didn't want to take my mom's freedom and privacy away. Not until it was absolutely necessary. I just didn't know when that would be.

To make matters worse, I laid alongside Mom worried that I'd done the wrong thing letting her go back to bed. What if she had a concussion? What if she fell asleep and never woke up?

What if something more serious was happening beneath the surface, more serious than a few minor bruises. I felt fairly confident she'd be okay, but what if she wasn't? What if I was wrong? I knew I'd never forgive myself if something happened to her.

The biggest question I struggled with that night was: Would any amount of safety measures keep her safe?

The following two weeks, Mom fell four more times. With each fall, I felt increasingly guilty that I wasn't there to prevent the situation. I was responsible for Mom's safety and well-being, but she kept getting hurt. One fall had even resulted in a broken rib. It was my job to care for her, and I was failing miserably. I decided the only way to prevent her from falling was to lay in bed with her until I could think of another option.

I asked my siblings for suggestions. How could we keep Mom safe? I'd noticed she slept on the edge of the mattress and I thought that might be the reason she'd fallen out of bed so many times, especially since the bed was so far off the ground. I suggested we consider purchasing an adjustable hospital bed that was closer to the ground. If she fell out of bed, she wouldn't fall far and hurt herself. We found a twin-size hospital bed for about two thousand dollars, but for only two hundred dollars we could buy bed rails for her queen-size bed. We considered the options, but I ultimately decided the rails were the better option. If the kids or I wanted to lie in bed with her to watch TV or comfort her, the rails would be easier to handle and afford us the room to lie next to her.

We also discussed the video monitor idea. I told my brothers and sister I was afraid of taking away Mom's freedom and privacy, but I also knew the baby monitor had been instrumental in how fast I'd found her when she'd fallen out of bed. After much discussion, we all agreed the video monitors would give us peace of mind, especially me since I was the one caring for Mom in my home. Ning immediately went to the store and bought two video monitors. We set them up so we could view the head and the foot of the bed. Although I still felt uneasy about installing the monitors, relief was the primary emotion. Knowing I could see what was going on with Mom any time she was in her room made me feel more at ease.

* * *

The nights I spent sleeping in Mom's room opened my eyes to the delusions she had at night. One night was particularly frightening when she insisted white mice were running across the ceiling. I assured her repeatedly that no mice were in her room, and no sooner had she settled down from that incident did she begin swinging her arm through the air trying to kill a roach that wasn't there. Then she began raising her hands upward, palms pushing toward the ceiling, convinced I was lying on top of her instead of next to her. At one point, she even insisted a family friend had climbed into bed with us.

After that night, I stopped sleeping in bed with her. I slept in the window seat instead. To say my nights were restless is an understatement. Between the discomfort of sleeping in the window seat and the hallucinations Mom had each night, I was exhausted times a million. I knew I couldn't continue to do this for the rest of Mom's life. Some nights, her hallucinations and delusions were so awful she'd throw things out of bed. One night, she thrashed about so much that she ended up sleeping with her head at the end of the bed.

Having the video monitors in her room and the bed rails made me feel better, but I knew it wasn't enough. If I was to work and raise my family without finding myself in an early grave, I needed more help. I hired a caretaker from church; we'll call her Annie. Over the course of Mom living with me, I hired many caretakers to help out, each with varying degrees of AD experience. Some were more helpful and trustworthy than others. One particular caregiver abused her and stole from us. It was a horrifying experience that made it difficult to trust any caregiver, and my experience with untrustworthy caregivers isn't unique. It's sad that there are people out there who only want to exploit families in need.

Annie had no experience with AD, but she did her best to care for Mom, and I appreciated her help. She came to our home Monday through Friday from noon to eight o'clock at night to help care for Mom. Annie was more than a babysitter. She was a blessing. Not only did she bathe and care for Mom, but she cleaned her room and washed her linens. Knowing I had someone in the house with Mom for eight hours each day while I was gone lifted so much weight from my shoulders. Annie and all the other caretakers that came in and out of our lives weren't the only help I had. Lauren helped too. She took care of her

Paw Paw from eight in the morning until noon. Kevin and I took care of her the rest of the time, ensuring she always had round-the-clock care. For the first time in a long time (or really ever), I felt like I had a handle on her care. Of course, AD likes to throw curveballs.

The first day Annie worked with Mom, she expressed concerns regarding her confusion, incoherency, and hallucinations. I was concerned too because she didn't recognize Kaden or me.

"Did your Mom fall recently?" she asked.

"She hasn't fallen for over a week. What do you think is wrong?"

"I'm concerned her symptoms could be a sign of a slow leak in her brain from a head injury."

We were already waiting for test results to see if Mom had a urinary tract infection (UTI), so when we called the doctor's office to check the status of those results, we asked if he wanted to see Mom to examine her for a possible head injury related to her last falling incident. Sometimes, when a UTI gets out of control, it can cause confusion, agitation, and combativeness in AD patients more so than other individuals because the pain and discomfort can amplify AD's symptoms. However, Mom's UTI test came back negative. Since we couldn't find a concrete cause for Mom's heightened confusion and disorientation, we took her to the emergency room right away.

Panic built up inside of me as I once again called the paramedics to come get Mom. Would the rest of her life be like this? Would we constantly call for ambulances to take her to the ER? What if she had a serious head injury? How would I forgive myself for letting this happen?

At the hospital, Mom underwent many tests, including blood work, a CAT scan of her brain, and X-rays. The doctors found nothing abnormal, other than slight dehydration. They gave Mom some fluids through an IV, and she began to perk up almost immediately. Her dehydration had simply added to the normal confusion that comes from having dementia. While older individuals are at a higher risk of dehydration, I learned that Alzheimer's patients have an even higher risk because they forget to drink throughout the day. As a caregiver to an Alzheimer's patient, the medical staff told me I needed to make sure Mom stayed well-hydrated. Not only did she need to drink more water, but adding specific foods to her diet, like ice cream, popsicles, fruit, vegetables, and soups, would help keep her hydrated. Every day I learned something more about what caring for an Alzheimer's patient meant, and it was a lot.

We spent a lot of time toward the end of Mom's life managing UTIs and dehydration and dealing with her doctors, who seemed like they wanted to write her off because she was in and out of the hospital so much. She had an incident nearly every other week that landed her in the hospital. The frustrating part about this process was how the doctors didn't seem to want to see Mom as anything more than a "textbook case" and not an individual. I spent so much time challenging her doctors because they didn't seem to want to treat her, the individual. They went straight to textbook diagnoses and answers, which never does patients any good because no two people are the same. There were times when the UTI went septic, prompting the doctors to speak with us about her quality of life. Whenever I heard the word *infection,* my heart and brain told me we could treat it and Mom would be okay. I reasoned that if Mom got sicker or the dementia started eating away at her brain, then I'd let her go peacefully.

We had Mom on hospice a handful of times based on the doctors' recommendations, but my level of care didn't wane; it only became more uncompromising while she was on hospice, and then she'd improve. So, she would be disqualified and removed from hospice. I knew Mom didn't need hospice care, but I relented because the doctors were insistent that the end was near. Thinking back on those times, I wish I hadn't surrendered to what the doctors thought was best because I knew Mom had more life in her.

Right now, as I write these words, I've been told that my sister-in-law, who has cancer and whom I take care of, needs hospital care. But she's doing better every day, regaining her strength and learning to walk again. The home healthcare nurses who come to the house to help with her care have said they believe she'll walk again and improve. She's not out for the count yet.

My point is this: Just because a doctor tells you to put your loved one in hospice doesn't mean it's the right thing to do if your heart feels it isn't. This is when you need to be an advocate for your loved one the most. I never felt like it was Mom's time each time she went into hospice, and because "no" isn't in my vocabulary, I worked extra hard to prove the doctors wrong and get her off of it. If you're reading this book and frustrated with the care your loved one's receiving, I want you to know it's okay to challenge doctors when you feel your loved one's being dismissed. It's okay to fight for your loved one.

When Mom came home from her latest hospital visit, her behavior toward Annie and subsequent caregivers became inconsistent. One moment she'd comply completely with requests, the next she'd get argumentative, especially when it came to bathtime. She often said she already bathed or that she didn't want any help. There were days when she'd barricade the door so Annie or no one else could get into her room, but when it was time for her to leave, Mom would hug her and say goodbye. She'd accuse caregivers of taking baths in her room or stealing from her, like she'd done to me and other members of the household. Sometimes, when Mom was being highly combative, she'd even threaten to call the police. When she got this agitated, I encouraged Annie or any of the other caregivers to walk away from Mom, drop the subject for a bit, and try again later. Putting some time and space between unwelcomed requests often was a great way to get Mom to bathe or eat because she'd forget about the arguments and be more agreeable.

Although most all the caregivers we had handled Mom's needs well, especially making sure she was fed and taking her medications, she called frequently to let me know what was happening. I was grateful for her concern, but I never got a moment of peace. Somedays, all I wanted was for complete silence and not having to put out fires all day long. I had no idea how long Mom would live with AD, and I'd hoped she'd outlast the doctors' expectations, but I also didn't know how long I could go on living in a constant state of uncertainty. How would Mom be today? What trouble would she get into, and would I be able to stop it before it happened?

***

The sound of the garage door opening at three in the morning one January day startled me awake. "Kevin," I whispered, shaking him gently awake, "did you hear that?"

"Hear what? What time is it?"

"It's three in the morning. Someone just opened the garage door. All the kids are in bed. Who would be coming home this late?"

"Are you sure you heard the garage door? Maybe you dreamt it?" I was wide awake by then and gave Kevin my most irritated wife look. He laughed and said, "Alright, let's go check it out."

We threw on our robes and treaded quietly down the hallway. All the bedroom doors were closed, so I couldn't tell if any of the kids had left their rooms. When we opened the interior door to the garage, we were startled. The garage door was wide open, and Mom was standing in bare feet on the driveway, with disheveled hair, wearing nothing but her nightgown. She looked as if she were searching for something.

I approached her slowly, like you would a wild animal, and said softly. "Mom, what are you doing out here?"

She turned to me, visibly upset.

"I'm looking for your father. I know he's out here somewhere." She sounded irritated. My heart broke hearing her speak those words. At that moment, she didn't remember Dad was gone. Should I remind her? No. I decided that would do more harm. Instead, I put my arm around her and guided her back into the house and got her settled in bed, surprised she didn't put up a fight.

While she slept, I sat in a chair by her bed, crying quietly so I wouldn't wake her. I felt so defeated. It didn't seem to matter what I did. Mom still escaped. She still put herself in danger unknowingly. What if she'd gone into the street and cut her feet on glass or other debris? What if something worse had happened, like she'd gotten hit by a car or wandered off and we couldn't find her? So many awful scenarios played through my mind like a horror-show montage. Would Mom one day end up on the news, a missing person? *Stop it,* I told myself. *You're doing your best. Go back to sleep. Mom is fine.* I went back to my bedroom, but I couldn't fall back asleep. I spent the rest of the early morning watching the video monitor while Mom slept.

Unfortunately, that night wouldn't be the last night Mom wandered. She wandered through the house most nights while the family slept. Several times, I'd catch her leaving the house in her nightgown, and each time frightened me more than the first. One day she left wearing nothing but her hospital gown, its back open and her backside exposed. She didn't make it further than our court. I spent so much time watching the video monitor waiting for her to leave her room that I got no sleep. When I asked her why she left her room, she usually said she was looking for my dad or her mother. She couldn't understand why she couldn't find them. A few times I tried to tell her they'd died, but that only upset her, and arguing with her only made things worse. So, I tried to redirect her or distract her with something else.

But Mom? Well, she had some elaborate explanations about where her late husband was. One time, she came out of her room dressed in street clothes with what she believed were car keys in her hands. I don't remember what she actually had in her hands—maybe some change or one of the kids' toys. All I remember is that it wasn't keys—thank God!

"I'm leaving," she announced.

"Where are you going?" I asked, playing along because sometimes it was just better to handle situations with Mom this way than trying to force my hand until it was absolutely necessary. Obviously, I wasn't going to let her get in the car.

"Your father has been living at that funeral home up the road and having an affair," she told me.

"What?" I stared at her incredulously. If she hadn't been so ill, it would've been humorous.

"He's having an affair, Bing, in that funeral home."

"Well, Mom, you're upset. So, how about I drive?"

I figured if I played along, she'd forget the delusion by the time we made it to the funeral home ten minutes up the road, but when I pulled into the parking lot, she said, "This isn't the one."

I wasn't going to drive all over town looking for the nonexistent funeral home my deceased dad was living at. I also wasn't sure how to go about getting Mom to understand Dad was gone and most certainly not having an affair. I suggested we go into the funeral home, hoping Mom would see for herself that what she thought was real wasn't. We got out of the car, walked into the funeral home, and since I moved faster than Mom, I made a quick beeline to the woman seated at the front desk.

"I'm so sorry to bother," I said to the woman in a hushed tone. "My Mom has Alzheimer's and thinks my dad, who died over ten years ago, is here. Can we walk around for a bit so I can show her he's not here?"

I admit, it was an insane thing to ask. I held my breath waiting for her response. The woman behind the desk was so kind to us. Not only did she let us walk around the building, she even played along when Mom asked for the number to the hospital where my father worked when he was alive. She gave my Mom the funeral home's number, probably not expecting that Mom would actually call it. Yet when we returned home, that's exactly what she did. Not only did she call the number, but she began speaking Cantonese thinking she was Dad's mistress.

Embarrassed, I took the phone from Mom and apologized profusely to the woman.

"I'm so sorry."

"Oh, honey, you don't have to apologize. I'm so sorry that you have to go through this. Good luck with everything."

I thanked her and hung up the phone. Turning back to Mom, I said, "Dad's working right now and really busy. He can't talk."

I expected an argument from her. Instead, she simply said okay, went to her room, and went to bed. I threw my hands in the air. *What just happened?* By then, I should've been used to Mom's antics, but Dad living at a funeral home with a mistress? At one point, Mom revisited the storyline she'd created and thought my brother's wife was at the funeral home having an affair with my dad. AD is such a convincing liar.

For a long while, Mom seemed hyperfocused on my dad's and grandmother's whereabouts. So I began making up stories about where they were to keep Mom from leaving the house. I would tell her Dad already left for work or Grandma went to the store. Sometimes the stories worked. Sometimes they didn't. When they didn't work, she'd wander outside in search for them, many times only in her nightgown. I couldn't predict when she'd believe the stories and when she wouldn't. Trying to keep her inside the house was exhausting. I worried constantly about her wandering off. The only solution I could come up with to keep her safe and stave off the constant worry was to install new locks on all the doors that required a PIN to unlock them. Once they were installed, I slept better at night.

Of course, the new security measures agitated Mom. She asked us all the time to unlock the doors. We pretended we didn't know how the locks worked. We weren't trying to gaslight Mom. We were only trying to keep her safe. The choices caregivers must make when caring for an AD patient seem cruel at times, but the loved one's safety must always come first. Unfortunately, Kevin took the brunt of Mom's frustration because she assumed he put the locks on the door. He took it in stride. No matter how many accusations she tossed his way, he always stood by my decision to care for Mom in our home. Even at her least lovable self, he continued to love and protect her at all costs. We all did.

Mom continued living with us for sixteen years after her initial probable Alzheimer's diagnosis, ten years longer than what her doctors told us she'd live. I have a million stories I could share, good and bad, and writing this memoir hasn't been easy at times. Thinking about the struggles we went through to make Mom's life and her end-of-life transition easier is difficult. The goals I had for Mom changed as the years went on. First, I wanted to prove she could thrive in our home and live longer than the doctors expected. Then, I wanted to get her the best care possible in our home, even when it became apparent that as one person, I couldn't do it all. And, finally, the goal was to get her to her ninetieth birthday. I didn't meet that last goal. Mom died on July 14, 2021, a little more than two months shy of her ninetieth birthday.

10

And Then It Was Over

Before Alzheimer's, Mom enjoyed spending time with her family, playing mahjong with her friends, and feeding the slot machines at the casinos. Her favorite thing to say was, "Go Vegas! Win money!" We got a kick out of listening to her hoot and holler while playing the slot machines—and could that woman play those machines! She won more than she lost. That's how I like to imagine her now, reveling in spiritual bliss among loved ones who passed on before her. I like to imagine she and my dad reunited. And although I no longer see her every day, I feel her presence, even more so as the years go on. People say time heals grief, but I'm not sure that's entirely true.

By the time this book is published, Mom will have been gone for over three years. Not a long time by any means, but long enough for life to fall back into a familiar groove. I stopped wearing black after the one-year anniversary and began wearing makeup again, two Chinese mourning traditions I followed. Yet grief's like a slow-dripping faucet; it exists in the background. We get used to it, finding a way to live with it the best we know how. Learning how to lay to rest the expectations we had for ourselves, our loved one, and our life. We get used to living with unanswered questions. But we never get over the loss.

After Mom passed, I didn't cry. The gut-wrenching sadness inside my body stayed buried deep inside, refusing to come out. That first year after Mom's death was about surviving all the "firsts": the first Christmas without her, the first Mother's Day, her first heavenly birthday. Learning how to live life with a little more breathing room, less caregiving, and fewer rigid schedules. Something I haven't mentioned until now is that I wasn't only caring for my mom. During the last few years of her life, I also provided care in my home for my cancer-stricken sister-in-law. So, while Mom no longer needed my care, my sister-in-law did. Perhaps caring for her created a sort of distraction from the grieving process. I don't know for sure. It took nearly a year before tears found their way down my cheeks and I tasted their saltiness on my tongue. Crying so hard I couldn't breathe.

After Mom passed, I wrote her this letter and put it in her casket:

Dearest Mommy,

I am going to miss you more than you will ever know. My mind tells me that you are in a better place, yet my heart is broken into a million pieces. You were my everything. You taught me how to be the greatest person I could be. For this, I will always thank you. You were the strongest person I ever knew. Please tell Dad hi. Please tell Oakley hi for Kameryn and all of us. I know over time my heart will heal some, but I will always and forever have you in my heart.

I love you!
Love Forever,
Bing

Why do we write letters to the dead? I can't speak for anyone reading this book, but for me, writing those words was cathartic. They released Mom and they released me—from what, I'm still not sure.

During the last four years of Mom's life, she became bedridden and completely dependent on myself and others for her care. We had to feed her and help her drink because she wouldn't and couldn't do it. One reason I've felt compelled to tell my story through writing and speaking is to help others feel less alone who find themselves caring for a loved one with AD or dementia. To do this effectively, it's important I don't sugarcoat the process. As Mom's AD battle began to wane, I did whatever I could to keep her with us for as long as possible. Yet she spent so much time the last year of her life in and out of the hospital that I'd be lying if I didn't question some of my decisions. Mom shared physical space with us, but she had been gone in all other ways for a long time. Her quality of life had diminished considerably.

One thing Mom did enjoy even as she neared the end was caring for her "babies." Mom had several baby dolls that she cuddled during the later stages of her disease. Witnessing Mom hold the baby dolls like they were living, breathing humans could trigger uncomfortable feelings, but eventually we welcomed the doll play. We came to see how doll play, which is a form of therapy for AD and dementia patients, helped Mom relax. It gave her pleasure and purpose. We also gave her a fidget blanket, similar to the activity blankets babies and toddlers use, with zippers, buttons, and various textures to help them learn. For Mom, the blanket kept her occupied. So did folding laundry. We would give Mom laundry over and over, often the same items like towels or shirts, to keep her busy. She never realized she was folding the same things again and again.

All the things we gave her to do to keep her happy and occupied often broke my heart, especially the dolls. Watching her care for the baby dolls reminded me of how much she had spoiled and doted on the twins when they were little.

It also made me incredibly sad because I knew Mom's time with us on earth was coming to an end—and I didn't know the best way to help her make that transition. I struggled with it happening at home or in the hospital. I didn't want her to die in the hospital, surrounded by machines and strange sounds. Yet I knew the possibility of her dying in the hospital was real. The last year of her life she'd been in the hospital at least every other week. She had a catheter to help her eliminate her bladder, which would give her painful urinary tract infections that would often go from zero to sixty, often turning septic. Each time Mom was admitted to the hospital, I stayed with her the entire time, even during the pandemic. I never left. How could I? Mom's English had completely left her, and her Chinese was pretty much done too as she'd become increasingly nonverbal.

Still, the thought of her dying in our home scared me too. If there's one thing I learned throughout the sixteen years I cared for Mom while she lived with AD, it's this: There are no easy decisions. Every decision has its benefits and its downsides.

Ultimately, Mom lost her battle with AD in the hospital surrounded by her family.

***

The last time Mom was admitted to the hospital, COVID-19 regulations were still in place. It was Sunday, July 11, 2021. Visitors were limited, no more than two at a time. Fortunately, the hospital staff waived these restrictions so the family could stay at Mom's side. Once we realized Mom wouldn't return home from this hospital stay, I remained suspended in a state of limbo and anxiousness. Although machines beeped and hummed in her room and the normal cacophony of hospital sounds played in the background, I didn't pay them much attention. Instead, I tried staying present, soaking in whatever moments I had left with my mom. I didn't shower. I wore the same outfit I had on the day the hospital admitted Mom. I slept in the room with her. I couldn't leave her side because I feared, in my absence, she'd take her last breath. I never left her side while she was in the ICU.

While she was in the hospital the last time, the doctor had put her on a BiPAP machine. The machine bought us some time for my siblings to get to the hospital to say their goodbyes. Mon traveled from California to St. Louis, the last to arrive on July 13. Caregiving is selfless, but if we're honest with ourselves, we also hope to control the outcome the best we can. Throughout Mom's life after Dad passed and her AD became increasingly problematic, I tried to control so much: her movements, living situation, her diet, her water intake, anything to make her comfortable, happy, and to keep her alive for as long as possible. With the end near, I had one more task, one final thing to control: I couldn't let Mom die on the thirteenth.

I'd never liked the number thirteen. There's no deep meaning behind my dislike of the number, nothing I can point a finger at and declare the reason thirteen makes my skin crawl. I simply didn't like it.

Also, the fourteenth had more meaning to me. In Cantonese, the number four, *sei* (pronounced say), means death. You've died. Keeping Mom alive until the fourth of August to get to that number wasn't an option. But I could keep her alive at least until *sahpsei* (sub day), the fourteenth of July. Again, the date a loved one dies seems arbitrary. I get it. But it mattered to me, and my family didn't argue. With everyone at the hospital, the doctors turned the BiPAP machine off just after midnight on July 14, 2021.

Mom kept us on our toes many times when she lived with us. And that wouldn't change as she transitioned to the other side. Once we turned the machine off, she didn't pass immediately. It would take some time, which gave us the time we needed for all the family to say goodbye. The family in town came to her room to say goodbye. Those who were out of town FaceTimed Mom to say their goodbyes.

After everyone had said their goodbyes, Lauren and Kameryn left. So did Kaden, but my girls decided to come back to the hospital to sit with Mom. While Lauren and Kameryn were at the hospital, Kaden called Kameryn to find out where she was. She explained she went back to the hospital, and Kaden decided he wanted to come back too, but it was after visiting hours. Lauren and Kameryn stepped out of Mom's room in the ICU to go get Kaden from the emergency room entrance. Shortly after they left, Mom took a huge breath and stopped breathing—her eyes wide open. I screamed at Wai, who was also in the room with me, to close her eyes. I called Kameryn, freaking out, and said, "She's gone! She's gone! You have to come back."

Kameryn told me later she turned away from Lauren in the hospital hallway as they were going to get Kaden, not even telling her what had happened, and ran as fast as her feet would carry her back to the room. When she made it back, her Paw Paw wasn't dead. Her breathing had restarted and she rested peacefully, waiting for Kaden to arrive. I feel like she knew he was on his way and waited for him because after my youngest son walked into Mom's room, she took her final breath. No curtain call or encore this time.

My mom, Kwai "Bessie" Chiu, died around 2:20 a.m. I don't remember the exact time. I'm sure I could look at her death certificate and find out that information, but I don't want to. I don't need the time etched in my brain. Some things are okay to let go.

After Mom passed, I wanted nothing more than to go home and sleep, but the aftermath of death requires so much work—more than you realize until it happens to you. Mon, Lauren,

Kameryn, and I stayed at the hospital with Mom until her transfer to the funeral home was completed. Mom passed on a Wednesday. We hoped to have her funeral that Friday or Saturday since Mon was already in town. But the funeral home couldn't accommodate our wishes because they had a full schedule. So, reluctantly, we took Mon to the airport and sent her back home.

I went home too and fell into one of the deepest sleeps of my life. While I slept, the funeral home tried to reach me to say they could accommodate our funeral services that weekend after all. It felt good to wake up to that news, but Mon was already on her way home. Fortunately, she and her family were able to fly back to attend the funeral. While Mon flew back, Ning and I made final arrangements at the funeral home. Thankfully, Mom had already made some arrangements for her funeral, including selecting her casket and floral arrangements.

The days leading up to the funeral were a blur for me. The thought of reaching out to everyone who needed to know about Mom's passing overwhelmed me. I figured the fastest and easiest way to do this was through social media. Work was the last thing on my mind at that moment, so I let my team handle informing my clients that Mom had passed away.

With social media handling the announcement and my team taking care of my clients, I had the space to manage the wake and funeral details, which by no means equaled an easy task. I had to put together the program, make picture boards, choose songs for the program, arrange for food at the wake and the funeral, and make "lucky envelopes."

In Chinese culture, funeral guests receive envelopes as they leave the ceremony. These little white envelopes include a piece of candy and a quarter. Guests eat the candy to add sweetness to the bitter occasion and spend the quarter before returning home to ward off bad spirits and pass good fortune on to others. To prepare the envelopes, we had to visit different banks to get rolls of quarters. Once we had all the quarters and candy, we set up an assembly line at the dining room table and got as much of the family as possible involved in putting quarters and candy in the little envelopes. We made over three hundred of these envelopes, but the funeral home didn't place them in a spot where everyone could see them. So, we ended up with many leftover envelopes. It made me sad that we were left with so many because putting together those envelopes was a part of Mom's Chinese culture and one last thing I could do for her in this life. My family and I took the quarters from the leftover envelopes and spent them at various places after the funeral. We weren't superstitious people, but we rolled with the tradition just to be on the safe side.

Mom's funeral was so beautiful. So many people stood up and spoke fondly of her, but none of that took away from how hard the day was for me. At the burial grounds, the casket slid from the metal framework while it was being lowered into the ground. I couldn't believe it! Luckily, the funeral staff corrected the issue quickly, and the burial continued. I don't think I'll ever forget what it was like to see the rainbow of colors on top of Mom's casket from the flowers thrown onto it by the funeral guests.

And then it was over.

I felt numb because that was it—the final part of Mom. I knew she no longer suffered, but my heart wouldn't receive the message. I wanted her back. I still do. Every single day I think of her and miss her, and that won't ever change until the day we're reunited.

LOVE, CARE, & ALZHEIMER'S

Epilogue

People often ask me if I fear getting Alzheimer's disease (AD). The short answer is yes, I fear it. In 2022, when I was fifty-five years old, I participated in a research study and had gene testing done to check for the AD gene. It took nearly nine weeks to get the results. The waiting game proved excruciating, and it didn't help that I'd been forgetting things. I probably had too much to remember; the forgetfulness was likely caused by stress and being overwhelmed. I'd been burning the candle at both ends for so long.

The genetic testing came back negative for the AD gene. What a relief! While it's still possible for me to have age-related dementia or nongenetic AD, knowing that it wasn't one hundred percent certain made me feel hopeful about the future.

After going through what I did caring for my mom, I knew I didn't want my children to bear that stressful and emotional toll. When I confessed my fears to my son, he half-jokingly told me he'd put me in the best nursing home. You might think I'd be upset hearing him say that, given how adamant I was about Mom not being in a nursing home, but you know what? I'm okay with that. I never want to burden my family.

Was caring for Mom a burden? Yes, at times, and at other times, it was a blessing. Still, I gave up so much of my life to care for her. Between working and caregiving, I wasn't always able to be there for my twins as much as I'd wanted. But caring for my mom gave me the chance to have a new relationship with her.

I never got an apology from Mom for how she turned away from the abuse I experienced as a child. We didn't have some Hollywood movie ending where the past mended itself through the caregiving process. I struggled with resentment and anger, but what I received was so much greater. I saw my mom as a human being, a person with struggles, vulnerabilities, and disappointment. Because, let's be honest, I gave up a lot of my life to care for her, but AD took even more from her: her memories, her independence, her ability to relate, and ultimately, her life.

If you're a caregiver to a loved one with AD or dementia, I honor your sacrifices. What you're doing is brutal, but to use a word made popular recently by the no. 1 *New York Times* bestselling author Glennon Doyle, it can also be "brutiful"—brutal and beautiful simultaneously.

What you're sacrificing for your loved one can't be measured. It's an experience no one wants, yet it's an experience unlike any other. Please don't forget to take care of yourself too. I didn't do a good job of that. I still struggle with caring for myself and putting my needs first. It's a work in progress, and as I write this book, I'm still caring for my sister-in-law. My greatest friend Ron, who has been a huge supporter of this book and of me telling my story, recently booked a cruise for us.

"You need to get away—and, no, you're not taking your computer," he told me.

I'm not used to others looking out for me. It's uncomfortable. I resist it often, but I'm starting to come around, my edges softening.

I hope you find softness in your life. Welcome help when it's offered. Ask for it when it's needed. You aren't alone.

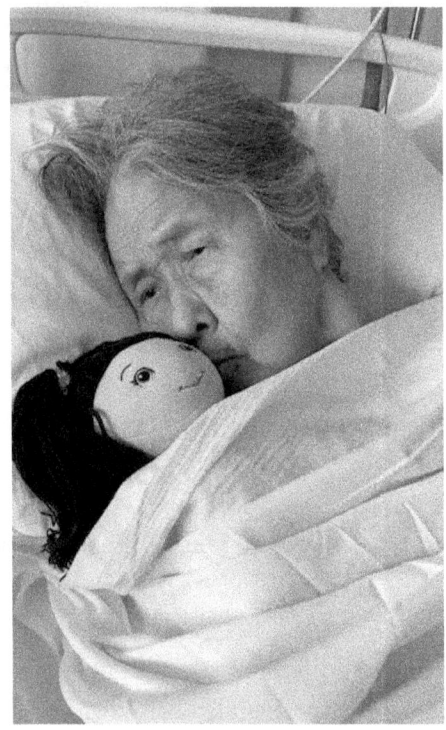

Mom and her doll.

Further Reading & Resources

Alzheimer's Society. "New research reveals one in three wait over a month to speak out about dementia worries." May 15, 2023. https://www.alzheimers.org.uk/news/2023-05-15/new-research-reveals-one-three-wait-over-month-speak-out-about-dementia-worries.

Wallensten, Johanna, Gunnar Ljunggren, Anna Nager, et al. "Stress, depression, and risk of dementia – a cohort study in the total population between 18 and 65 years old in Region Stockholm." *Alzheimer's Research & Therapy* 15, no. 161 (2023). https://doi.org/10.1186/s13195-023-01308-4.

Willis, Tallulah, and Rob Haskell. "Tallulah Willis on Grief, Healing, and the Road Ahead." *Vogue*, May 31, 2023. https://www.vogue.com/article/bruce-willis-and-me-memoir-tallulah-willis.

World Health Organization (WHO). "Dementia." March 15, 2023. https://www.who.int/news-room/fact-sheets/detail/dementia.com

About the Author

Bing Dempewolf is the founder and CEO of TAI-CHI Consulting, a professional HR company focused on helping veterans transition to the civilian workforce, students develop work-related experiences that complement their education, workers in transition receive career coaching and counseling, and disadvantaged workers reenter the job market. She is also the board president of The Women's Safe House in St. Louis and a board member of the St. Louis Society for the Blind and Visually Impaired. When she's not working or volunteering with community organizations, she enjoys spending time with her family and advocating for Alzheimer's and dementia patients, as well as supporting their caregivers. *Love, Care & Alzheimer's: A Daughter's Memoir* is her first book.

www.ingramcontent.com/pod-product-compliance
Lightning Source LLC
Chambersburg PA
CBHW071719020426
42333CB00017B/2323